JOHN EBNEZAR CBS | Handbooks in Orthopedics and Fractures

SERIES

Orthopedic Trauma

Sports Injuries

Volume I

- Sports Injuries
- Soft Tissue Injuries in Sports
- Upper Limb Injuries in Sports

John Ebnezar

- Holder of the **Guinness Book of World Records** for the most number of books written by an individual in a single year.
- Listed in the **India Book of Records** for the most number of books written by an individual.
- Recipient of the highest civilian awards of Karnataka, the **Rajyotsava Award 2010** and the **Kempegowda Award 2011**.
- Recipient of the **Best Citizen of India Award** by the International Publishing house.
- Former Vice-President, the Indian Orthopaedic Association
- President, Neuro-Spinal Surgeons Association of India (Karnataka)
- CEO, Parimala Health Care Services, A ISO 9001:2008 Hospital, Bilekahalli, Bannerghatta Road, Bangalore
- Ebnezar Orthopedic Center, Bilekahalli, Bannerghatta Road, Bangalore
- Dr John's Orthopedic Clinic, near Reliance Mart, Arakere, BG Road, Bangalore
- Chairman, the Physically Handicapped and Paraplegic Charitable Trust of Karnataka®
- Founder President, Geriatric Orthopedic Society
- Founder President, Orthopedic Authors Association and All India Medical Authors Association
- Chairman, Karnataka Orthopedic Academy®
- President, Bangalore Holistic Academy
- Chairman, Rakesh Cultural Academy
- President, Vaidya Kala Ranga, Bangalore
- Secretary, SK Educational Society®
- Former Senior Specialist, Victoria Hospital, Bangalore Medical College, Bangalore
- Former Assistant Professor in Orthopedics, Devaraj Urs Medical College, Kolar, Karnataka
- Postgraduate teacher, Bangalore Baptist Hospital, Airport Road, Bangalore

John Ebnezar CBS | Handbooks in Orthopedics and Fractures

SERIES

Orthopedic Trauma

Sports Injuries

VOLUME I

- Sports Injuries
- Soft Tissue Injuries in Sports
- Upper Limb Injuries in Sports

John Ebnezar

MBBS, D'Ortho, DNB (Ortho), MNAMS (Ortho), PhD (Yoga)
Sports Medicine (Australia), INOR Fellow (UK), DAc, DMT

Consulting Orthopedic and Spine Surgeon,
Holistic Orthopedic Expert, and Sports Specialist
Bangalore

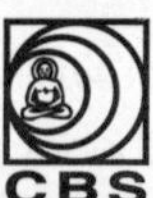

CBS Publishers & Distributors Pvt Ltd

New Delhi • Bengaluru • Pune • Kochi • Chennai

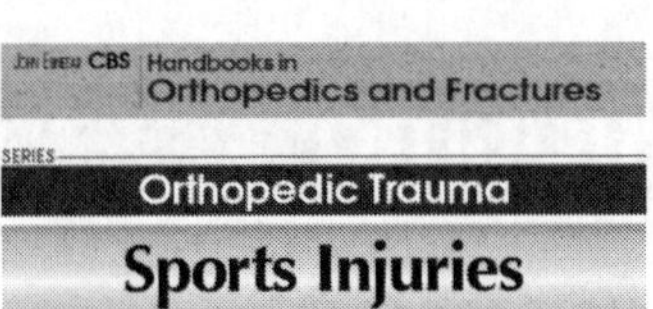

VOLUME I

ISBN: 978-81-239-2101-3

First Edition: 2012

Published by Satish Kumar Jain and produced by Vinod K. Jain for
CBS Publishers & Distributors Pvt Ltd
4819/XI Prahlad Street, 24 Ansari Road, Daryaganj
New Delhi 110 002, India.
Ph: 23289259, 23266861, 23266867
Fax: 011-23243014
Website: www.cbspd.com
e-mail: delhi@cbspd.com
cbspubs@airtelmail.in.

Branches

- Bengaluru: Seema House 2975, 17th Cross, K.R. Road, Banasankari 2nd Stage, Bengaluru 560 070, Karnataka
  Ph: +91-80-26771678/79 Fax: +91-80-26771680 e-mail: bangalore@cbspd.com
- Pune: Bhuruk Prestige, Sr. No. 52/12/2+1+3/2 Narhe, Haveli (Near Katraj-Dehu Road Bypass), Pune 411 051, Maharashtra
  Ph: 020-64704058, 64704059, 32392277 Fax: +91-020-24300160 e-mail: pune@cbspd.com
- Kochi: 36/14 Kalluvilakam, Lissie Hospital Road, Kochi 682 018, Kerala
  Ph: +91-484-4059061-65 Fax: +91-484-4059065 e-mail: cochin@cbspd.com
- Chennai: 20, West Park Road, Shenoy Nagar, Chennai 600 030, Tamil Nadu
  Ph: +91-44-26260666, 26208620 Fax: +91-44-45530020 email: chennai@cbspd.com

Printed at Magic International, Greater Noida (UP)

to

---

my mother
(late) Sampath Kumari
who taught me that life is more than self and
there is more joy in giving and sharing than taking

my wife
Dr Parimala

my lovely children
Rakesh and Priyanka
who are an epitome of love, sacrifice, encouragement
and inspiration

all my teachers
who made me what I am today

all my students
past and present

and

all my patients

Dr John Ebnezar

is a legendary name as a prolific orthopedic writer. No other orthopedic surgeon in the world has come anywhere close to him in the number of books he has written in his field. He is the first orthopedic surgeon in the world to be listed in the **Guinness Book of World Records** for the most number of books written by an individual in a single year. For the same feat his name has been listed in the **India Book of Records.** This book, like all his previous books, carries his flavor of simple and lucid writing, excellent language, beautiful illustrations and excellent presentation of the topics. This book is a part of the 100+ book series he has brought out in a single calendar year of 2012 on a wide array of orthopedic problems of public health importance. No other individual in the world has brought out these many books in one year and this is a world record attempt. With these books he aims to educate the reader and the public about these common orthopedic problems.

All his books have been accepted very well and he has a great fan following all over the world. He has been bestowed with as many as 32 international, national and state awards including Karnataka state's highest civilian award the **Rajyotsava Award 2010** and the **Kempegowda Award 2011,** apart from the **Best Citizen of India Award** given by the International Publishing House. He is the pioneer in holistic orthopedics and is credited for discovering a new method of treatment for the common orthopedic problems and has done PhD in arthritis from the world famous S-VYASA University, Bangalore. He is currently president of the Neuro-Spinal Surgeons Association of India (Karnataka), the former Vice-President of the Indian Orthopedic Association, and is the founder president of various orthopedic bodies.

Preface

This book is a part of the 100+ book series

JOHN EBNEZAR CBS Handbooks in Orthopedics and Fractures

which deals with the orthopedic problems of public health importance. The purpose of these books is to educate and create awareness among the readers about various problems associated with orthopedics. Through this way the readers get to know all about various orthopedic problems directly from a specialist. This will help a reader immensely in getting the right knowledge as most of them depend on the internet and magazines which distort and misrepresent various pieces of information concerning health topics, leaving the readers confused and worse still improperly educated. This may harm more than helping them find solutions to their problems. The purpose of these books, therefore, is to educate the readers right in their quest for knowledge on the common health and associated problems.

The 100+ book series has been brought out in a single calendar year.

Sports as a career is being considered by a vast majority of people in recent times It is no more a taboo as a profession thanks to the encouragement, support earning opportunities and fame associated with most of the sports like cricket, tennis, badminton, athletics etc. As more and more people are taking up sports, sports related problems are on the rise. Among the various sports related problems, orthopedic injuries associated with sports are seeing an increasing trend. Orthopedic related sports injuries can range from a minor strain to sprain or to a major fracture and dislocation of any of the bone or joints. Diagnosis and managing them is quite a challenge as unlike in a general population, a sportsperson needs to get back to the sporting action fast. For this to happen, diagnosis and treatment have to be perfect and most importantly the rehabilitation program has to be very good. The career of a sportsman is short and any error or mismanagement of sports related orthopedic injury can prematurely cut short their professional life. Hence it is of paramount important to tackle sports related injuries effectively. This book enables the reader to have a glimpse about all the issues related to sports injuries. As with all the books in these series, this book also aims to educate the reader and create awareness about sports related orthopedic injuries.

This is the first ever book which exclusively deals with the orthopedic sports injuries and I have made an attempt to bring all the important basic aspects about it in one book, so that the reader gets to know about them.

Highlights of this book

- Simple and lucid language
- Good illustrations
- Good clinical photographs wherever necessary
- Relevant X-rays
- Short summaries
- Anecdotes

This book has ubiquitous utility and usage and can be useful to the orthopedic surgeons, postgraduate students in orthopedics, undergraduate medical students, doctors from all disciplines of medicine, physiotherapists, therapists practising alternative systems of medicine, rehabilitation specialists, and most importantly the common people. It is particularly useful to those unsung heroes who work in remote areas with minimum infrastructure. They can use this book as a ready-reckoner. Seldom will you find a book that covers such a wide spectrum of readers.

Knowing all about the sports injuries creates awareness and helps one to understand them well and thereby prevent complications from happening.

Constructive criticism and useful suggestions are invited to make the book more effective in its forthcoming editions.

John Ebnezar

Acknowledgments

This volume is a part of the 100+ book series brought out in a single calendar year. This was a huge and mammoth task attempted first time ever by an author and a publisher in the world. Such an herculean effort could not have been possible without the active involvement of those concerned in CBS Publishers & Distributors. I thank Mr Satish K Jain, Managing Director of CBS P&D, for agreeing to be a part of this world-record feat in bringing out this book in the Series. My special thanks to Mr YN Arjuna who showed special interest in this work and channelized his entire energy into this improbable feat. My special thanks to Mrs Ritu Chawla and her entire dedicated team who have toiled day and night to make this dream a reality. I thank members of the entire editorial–production team of CBS P&D who have worked hard behind the scenes to bring out this book.

My special thanks to Dr Yogitha for actively helping me in the compilation of all the books. I also thank all the staff members of my hospital who have helped me at various levels during the making of this book.

John Ebnezar

Contents

JOHN EBNEZAR **CBS** | Handbooks in

Orthopedics and Fractures

TITLES IN THE SERIES

I Orthopedic Trauma

General Fractures

1 General Principles of Fractures and Dislocations
2 Fracture Treatment Methods
3 Fractures and their Complications
4 Atypical Fractures

Injuries of Upper Limb

5 Injuries of Shoulder
6 Injuries of Arm
7 Injuries of Elbow
8 Injuries of Forearm
9 Injuries of Wrist and Hand
10 Injuries of Distal Forearm and Wrist
11 Injuries of Hand
12 Injuries of Upper Limb

Injuries of Lower Limb

13 Injuries of Hip
14 Injuries of Femur
15 Injuries of Knee
16 Injuries of Knee and Leg
17 Injuries of Ankle and Leg
18 Injuries of Ankle and Foot
19 Injuries of Lower Limb

Injuries of Axial Skeleton

20 Injuries of Pelvis and Hip
21 Injuries of Spine
22 Injuries of Pelvis and Spine

23 Sports Injuries Vol I
24 Sports Injuries Vol II
25 Soft Tissue Problems in Orthopedics
26 Geriatric Trauma
27 Pediatric Trauma

II Orthopedic Disease

28 Congenital Orthopedic Problems
29 Developmental Orthopedic Problems

III Specific Orthopedic Problems

IV Regional Orthopedic Problems

V Orthopedic Injuries and Surgeries

VI Practical Examination

VII Orthopedic Problems of Different Ages

VIII Common Orthopedic Problems

IX Yoga Therapy in Common Orthopedic Problems

1 Sports Injuries

Introduction

Our cricketing icons; master blaster Sachin Tendulkar, ace spinner Anil Kumble, Nawab of Najafgarh Virender Sehwag, the effervescent VVS Laxman and the rock of Gibraltar Rahul Dravid, Sree Shanth all were in the news for sports injuries. For once, these injuries outfamed and outshone these cricketing demigods and were discussed and talked by everyone than the cricketers themselves. Therefore, these injuries fall within the gambit of sports medicine, which is in fact a developing science with tremendous potential. With more and more people taking up sports as a career, the sports-related injuries are on the rise.

Sports medicine, like all other branches of medicine, aims at the complete physical, mental and spiritual well-being of a sportsperson. A healthy mind in a healthy body is a concept, which is more true to a sportsperson than anybody else. Positive thinking, fairplay and sportsmanship should be the hallmark of a true sportsman. We, the doctors and the therapists, aim to keep a sportsperson physically fit so that the rest of the objectives mentioned above are attained automatically.

Like in other branches of medicine so in sports medicine, prevention is better than cure. To prevent sports injuries, the first step is to ascertain whether a person choosing sports is fit to take it. An unfit person taking up sports is a sure prescription for future sports injuries. A fitness testing for those who wish to take up sports as their career should include various relevant parameters (see box).

Quick facts: Sports vs fitness testing

- Muscle power should be adequate.
- Active joint movements.
- Range of passive movements.
- Body balance.
- Coordination skills.
- Symmetrical and coordinated movements between the limbs and the body.
- Elasticity and extensibility of muscles and ligaments.
- Presence of any unwanted or accessory movements.

These and many other factors determine whether a person is fit enough to take to sports.

However, one has to remember that fitness testing is not done only at the initial stages but needs to be done repeatedly at every stage of an athlete or a sportsperson's life. The second stage of prevention of sports-related injuries is assessing whether a sportsman is fit enough to resume the sporting activity after the initial layoff. There is nothing more dangerous than an unfit or a partially fit person resuming the sporting activity. It may spell a doom to his otherwise flourishing career in sports. A sportsperson has to satisfy certain norms before he can finally be sent back to the field (see box).

Quick facts

A sportsperson has to satisfy the following norms before he resumes sports:

- Should be able to jump from a height of 1 meter.
- Full range of painless active movements.
- Slight pain at extreme movements against resistance.
- No running limp.
- Can fully squat with one or both legs.
- Can do full press up.
- Can extend the knee with 20 lb × 10 in 45 sec.

- Persons engaged in contact sports should be able to lift 45 lb × 10 in less than 45 sec.
- The sportsperson should be independent of any strapping or support.

If a person satisfies all the above criteria, he can be safely returned back to his passion, i.e. sports.

CLASSIFICATION OF SPORTS INJURIES

Among the various classifications proposed for sports injuries, the one proposed by Williams (1971) is widely used and recommended.

Williams' Classification

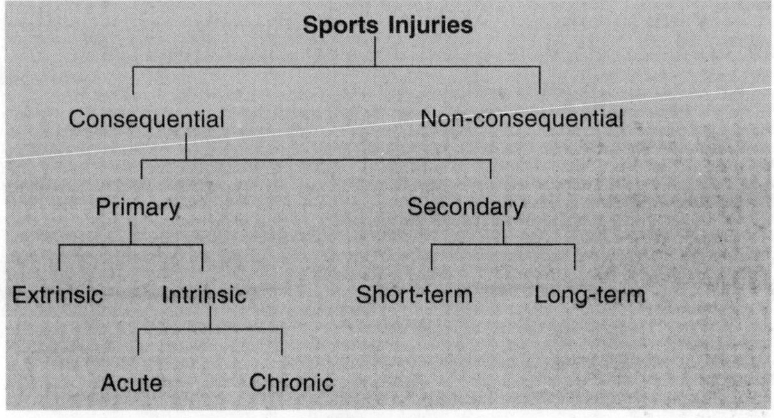

Among the Consequential Injuries

Primary Extrinsic

This is further subdivided into:

- *Human:* Black eye due to direct blow.
- *Implemental:* May be incidental (as in blow from a hard ball) or due to overuse (blisters from oars).
- *Vehicular:* Clavicle fracture due to fall from cycle, etc.
- *Environmental:* Injuries in divers.
- *Occupational:* Jumper's knee in athletes, chondromalacia in cyclists, etc.

Primary Intrinsic

This could be acute or chronic.

- *Incidental:* Strains, sprains, etc.
- *Overuse:*
  - Acute, e.g. acute tenosynovitis of wrist extensors in canoeists.
  - Chronic, march fracture in soldiers, etc.

Secondary

Short-term: For example, quadriceps weakness.
Long-term: Degenerative arthritis of the hip, knee, ankle, etc.

Non Consequential Injuries

These are not related to sports but are due to injuries either at home or elsewhere and are very not connected to any sports (e.g. slip and fall at home).

COMMON SPORTS INJURIES

Sports medicine usually deals with minor orthopedic problems like soft tissue trauma (Fig. 1.1). Very rarely, there may be serious fractures, head injuries or on the field deaths (Fig 1.2), especially in high speed contact sports. There is nothing unusual about these injuries except that a sportsperson demands a 100 percent cure and recovery while an ordinary person is satisfied and happy with a 60–80 percent recovery. The difference is because of the desire of the sportsperson to get back to the sport again, which requires total fitness.

> *Note*: The incidence of sports injuries among all orthopedic injuries is 5–10 percent.

The following are some of the most common sports-related injuries one encounters in clinical practice.

Upper Limbs

- *Shoulder complex*
  - Rotator cuff injuries

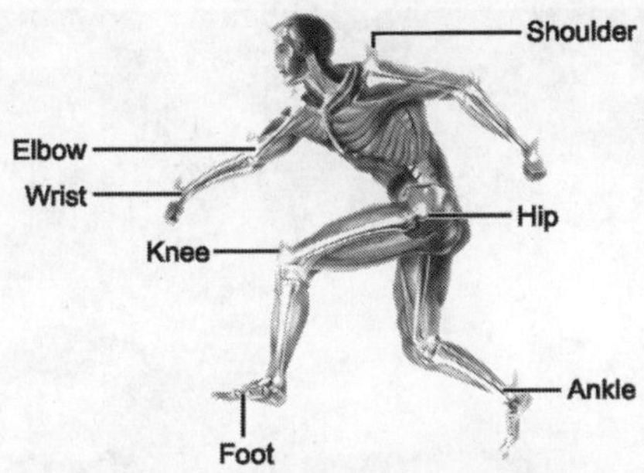

Fig. 1.1: Common sites of soft tissue injuries in sports

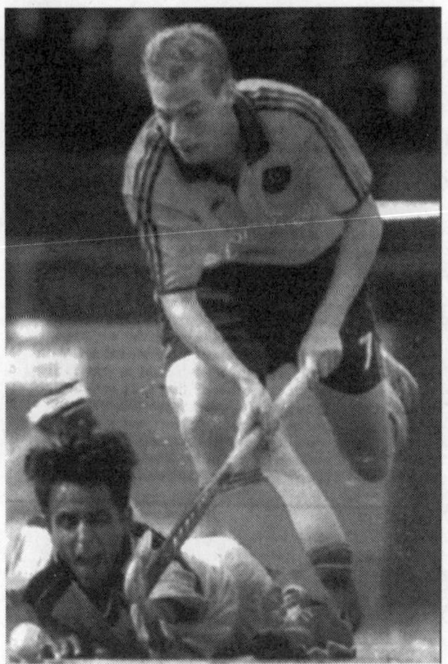

Fig. 1.2: Frequent falls, contact injuries and high-speed activities are the common causes of sports injuries

- Shoulder dislocations
- Fracture clavicle
- Acromioclavicular injuries
- Bicipital tendinitis or rupture.

- *Elbow*
  - Tennis elbow (Fig. 1.3)

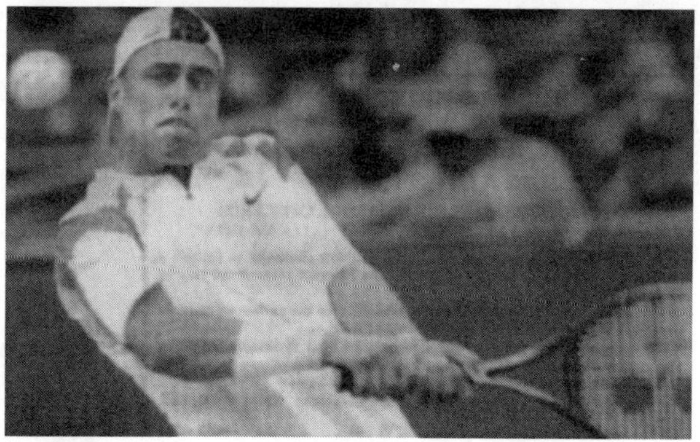

Fig. 1.3: Professional tennis players most commonly suffer from a famous sports disorder tennis elbow

  - Golfer's elbow
  - Dislocation of elbow.
- *Wrist*
  - Wrist pain
  - Carpal tunnel syndrome.
- *Hand*
  - Mallet injury (Fig. 1.4)
  - Baseball finger

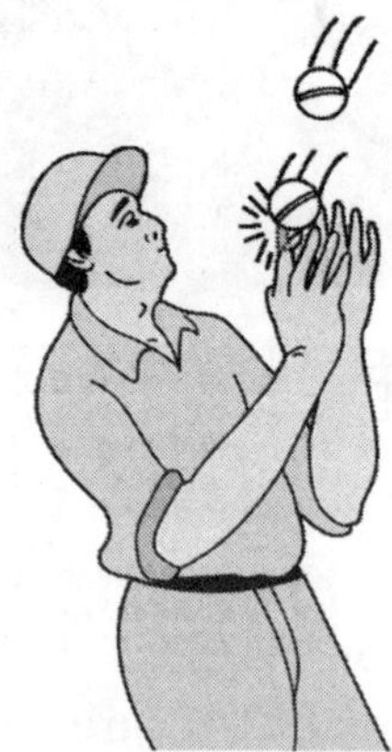

Fig. 1.4: Mechanism of mallet finger injuries in cricketers while trying to catch a ball

  - Jersey thumb
  - Injuries to the finger joints.

Lower Limbs

- *Hip*
  - Iliotibial or tract syndrome
  - Quadriceps strain
  - Hip pain
  - Groin pain due to adductor strain.
- *Knee Joint*
  - Jumpers knee
  - Chondromalacia
  - Fracture patella
  - Knee ligament injuries
  - Meniscal injuries.
- *Legs*
  - Calf muscle strain
  - Hamstrings sprain
  - Stress fracture tibia
  - Compartmental syndrome of the leg.
- *Ankle Injuries*
  - Ankle sprain
  - Injuries to tendo-Achilles
  - Tenosynovitis.
- *Foot*
  - March fracture
  - Jones fracture
  - Forefoot injuries
  - Injuries of sesamoid bone of the great toe.

Head, Neck, Trunk and Spine

- Head injuries
- Whiplash injuries
- Rib fractures
- Trunk muscle strains

- Abdomen muscle strain
- Low backache
  All these injuries have been discussed in relevant sections.

Investigations

These are the same as for any orthopedic-related disorders and consists of plain X-ray, CT scan, bone scan, MRI, arthroscopy, arthrography, stress X-rays, etc.

TREATMENT OF SPORTS INJURY

This is discussed under three headings: prevention, proper treatment and training.

Preventive Measures

The best way to treat a sports injury is to prevent it from happening. Nothing is better than preventing the injury.

Treatment

Treatment of individual sports-related disorders is discussed under suitable sections. However, a mention is made here

Quick facts

Preventive measures

- Proper clinical examination to identify any bodily defects.
- Fitness training.
- Correcting the wrong body mechanics and posture.
- Conditioning exercises to overcome particular deficiencies.
- Cardiopulmonary conditioning exercises to develop endurance.
- Proper warm up exercises and relaxation techniques before and after the sports.
- Wearing proper footwears and other protective devices like helmet, gloves, etc.
- To prevent overuse syndrome, taking adequate breaks in between the vigorous sports is advised.
- Avoiding sports in very high or low temperature climates.
- Not allowing aggravating minor problems like contusion, sprain, etc. by taking adequate rest and treatment.

of the general principles of treatment which is applicable to all sports injuries.

General Principles

- *Concept of RICEMM:* This sums up the early treatment methodology of sports injuries and consists of:
  R — Rest to the injured limb
  I — Ice therapy
  C — Compression bandaging
  E — Elevation of the injured part
  M — Medicines like painkillers, etc.
  M — Modalities like heat, straps, supports, etc.
- After immobilization and rest, early vigorous exercises should be commenced at the earliest to prevent muscle weakness and atrophy.
- To prevent joint stiffness, early mobilization has to be done first by passive movements and later by active movements. To improve the strength, resistive exercises are added.
- Unlike the conventional once a day treatment, a sportsperson needs to be seen at least 2–3 times a day.
- As mentioned earlier, allow resumption of sporting activity only after the sportsperson assumes 100 percent fitness.
- Mind training is as important as physical training. By repeated counseling, improve the psychological status of the patient to avoid depression, anxiety and negative attitudes, which may develop during the injury.
- Orthopedic and surgical treatment to be undertaken at appropriate situations.

Training

The physiotherapist has to train a sportsperson in various exercises to enable him to keep his fitness level very high. After conducting a fitness testing (mentioned earlier), the therapist has to subject an athlete to various forms of exercises to increase the endurance, strength, running, weightbearing, etc. The following are the various forms of exercises.

Exercises to Increase the Cardiopulmonary Capacity

These exercises are done to increase the endurance level of an athlete or sportsperson.

Exercises to Increase the Muscle Strength

By carefully planned, graded, progressive resistive exercises (PRE), the therapist aims at improving the strength of the muscles of the upper limbs, lower limbs, trunk and spine.

Quick facts: PRE (Progressive Resistive Exercises)

- For upper limb muscles—bench press
- For lower limb muscles—squatting exercises
- For trunk and muscles of the limbs—power clean.

Exercises for Free Weight Training

Strength training with machines has a disadvantage in training only the prime movers. This anomaly is converted by free weight training, which helps to strengthen not only the prime movers but also the synergistic and stabilizing groups of muscles (e.g. exercises with dumb bells). They are also known to increase the tensile strength of the muscles, ligaments and tendons.

Measures to Improve the Agility

The measures to improve the agility levels of sportsperson are two-leg hops, one-leg hop, cross over-run turning, bending and backward running. These exercises help to improve balance, coordination and movements at a faster rate.

Measures to Improve the Speed-polymetrics

In this, the neuromuscular system is trained to such an extent that it can react very quickly to sudden increase of speed and power, which is so often required in sporting activities.

Measures of Relaxation

After the vigorous workout mentioned above, the sportspeople are taught methods of relaxation and body stretches.

Quick facts: About polymetrics

- Hops
- Speed jumps
- Running drills
- These above exercises must be done very fast with sudden burst of energy.
- The speed strength of a sportsperson depends on how fast the muscle action changes from eccentric to concentric ones.
- This is then followed with graded resistance exercises.

Before an athlete or a sportsperson resumes his sporting activities, a fitness testing is carried out and only then, he is allowed to take to the sports provided if he is 100 percent fit.

BIBLIOGRAPHY

1. Bass AL. Rehabilitation after soft tissue injury. Proceedings of the Royal Society of Medicine, 653–56.
2. Fowler JA. Fitness and its components. Physiotherapy, 63.
3. Hornor Z, Werpravnik C. Mechanisms, types and treatment of injuries. British Journal of Sports Medicine, 1: 45–46.
4. Williams JGP. Classification of Sports Injuries, 1971.
5. Wright D. Fitness testing after injury. In Reilly T (Ed): Sports Fitness and Sports Injuries. London: Faber and Faber.

2 Soft Tissue Injuries in Sports

Introduction

Soft tissue injuries are not quite 'soft' but 'hard' in terms of management and rehabilitation. The term soft tissue implies skin, subcutaneous tissue, fascia, muscles, ligaments, tendons, synovium, capsules, nerves, etc. (Fig. 2.1). Undoubtedly, they are more common than bony injuries. Sportspeople are more prone to suffer from soft tissue injuries than the normal population. Unlike in fractures, the

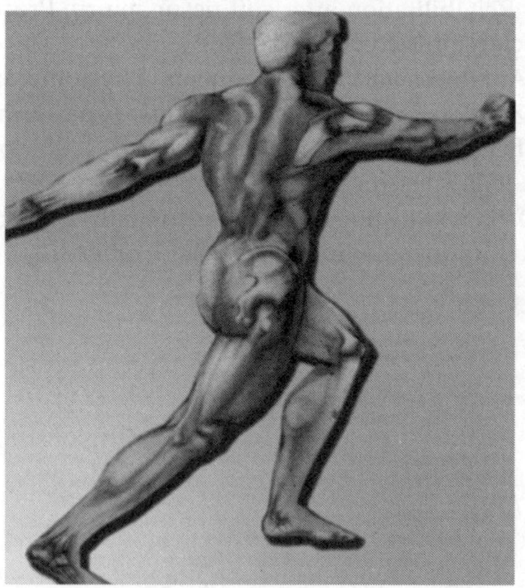

Fig. 2.1: Sites of common soft tissue injuries

soft tissue injury management is essentially conservative and physiotherapy appears to be the mainstay of treatment.

Mechanism of Injury

Direct Trauma

Due to fall, RTA, assault, etc. Contusion, hematomas, lacerations are some of the examples.

Indirect Trauma

Due to avulsion injuries, muscle pull, ligament sprain, etc. More commonly seen in sportspeople.

Approach to a Patient with Soft Tissue Injury

The Patient's Story

Listen to what the patient has to say about the problem. Do not be swayed by his story. He may be going overboard. Take his complaints with a 'pinch of salt'. This is the subjective assessment.

Your Observation

This is your assessment of the problem based on 'his' story. Make an objective assessment of the injury with regard to site, nature, intensity of pain, etc. of the injury. Your evaluation may or may not co-relate with 'his' story. Evaluate carefully the functional problem, interpret it analytically and individualize the treatment plan.

Goal Setting

A surgeon needs to set-up goals while treating soft tissue injuries. These could be immediate or long-term.

Execution of Your Plan

Having made a careful evaluation of the injury; you have sized up the problem and formulated your modus operandi. Keeping both the short and long-term goals in mind unleash your plan of action now to bottle up this genie.

Treatment Goals of Soft Tissue Injury

Immediate Goals

This aims to 'nip' the problem in the bud and 'prevent' further damages from taking place. A look at the priorities clarifies this:

- If there is blood loss—arrest it, prevent it, control it.
- If there is swelling—try to minimize it.
- If there is pain—try to alleviate it.
- If there is joint stiffness—try to prevent it.
- In all possibility try to see that there is no further damage whatsoever once you are in charge of the injury.
- In the event of muscle weakness—try to maintain the power.

Thus, immediate goals aim at 'prevention' of further damage and injuries to the soft tissues.

The Distant Goals

Here your efforts are to put the derailed life of the soft tissues back on rails and restore the structures to their pre-injury state. No mean task this and it calls for a sustained and skillful approach. The priorities in this are as under:

- *Movements:* Restore it to as normal as possible.
- *Mobility:* Ensure the affected joints are back to their best.
- *Strength:* The affected muscles need to be given their strength and endurance back.
- *Kinesthetic/proprioception mechanism:* Restore it back to normal.
- *Daily or functional activities:* Restore it back to the original.
- *Confidence:* Boost the patient's morale and that of the affected part.
- *Keep away:* The swelling, edema from raising its ugly head again. Once bitten twice shy, hence no more such injuries.
- *Last but not the least:* Ensure that this problem will not surface again by practicing effective anti-recurrent methods.

- *Inculcate:* A sense of discipline in practicing regular follow-up and valuing the medical advice. Drive home the advantages of 'home care' programs. Instill in them a thought that, "it pays to be your own doctor in the safe confines of their home".

Classification of Soft Tissue Injury

The four broad classifications for STI are as follows:
- Strains
- Sprains
- Ruptures
- Contusions.

Let us now discuss each one in detail.

MUSCLE INJURY (STRAINS)

Definition

Injury to the muscle and tendons is called *strain* (Fig. 2.2).

Reasons

- Sudden unaccustomed or abrupt action or movements may tear the muscles.
- Direct trauma can also injure the muscles and tendons.

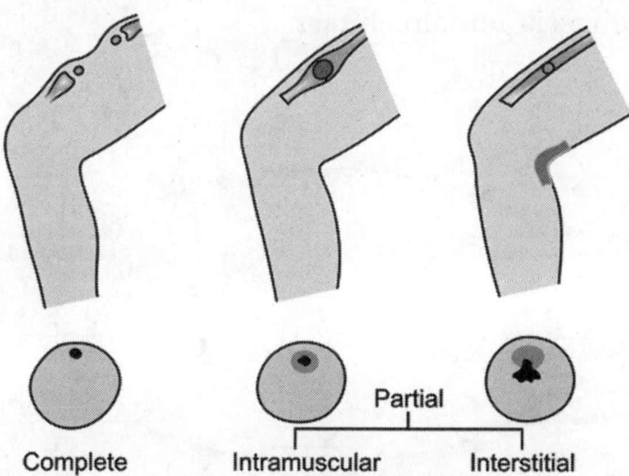

Fig. 2.2: Types of muscle strains

- Overstretching of muscles due to indirect trauma, especially in sportspeople.

Types

Acute strain: This is due to sudden violent force or direct trauma.
Chronic strain: This is due to injury existing since a long period leading to muscle ischemia and fibrosis.

Pathophysiology

Injury to the muscles leads to pain. As a result, the muscle goes into spasm to limit the movements and reduce pain. Nevertheless, paradoxically, this protective muscle spasm causes pain due to stimulation of pain fibers and thus a vicious cycle sets in Fig. 2.3. The painful stimuli cause muscle spasm through the peripheral nociceptive stimuli (Fig. 2.4).

Severity of Strain

Grade I

First Degree Strain (Mild Contusion)

- This is due to blunt injury and is due to direct trauma of low intensity.
- *Pathology:* Few muscle fibers are torn. Bleeding is minimal and the fascia remains intact.

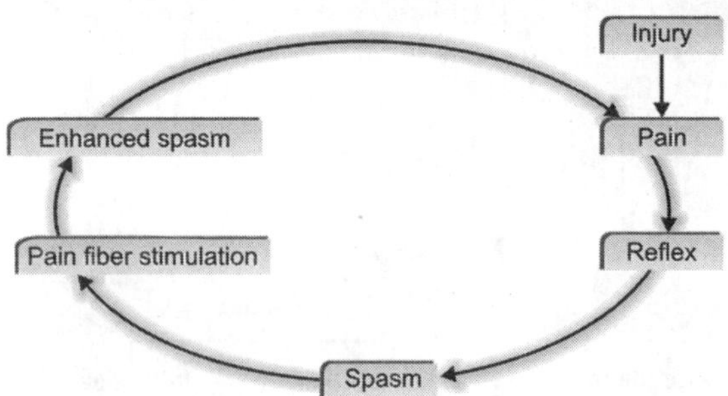

Fig. 2.3: Pain and spasm: The vicious cycle

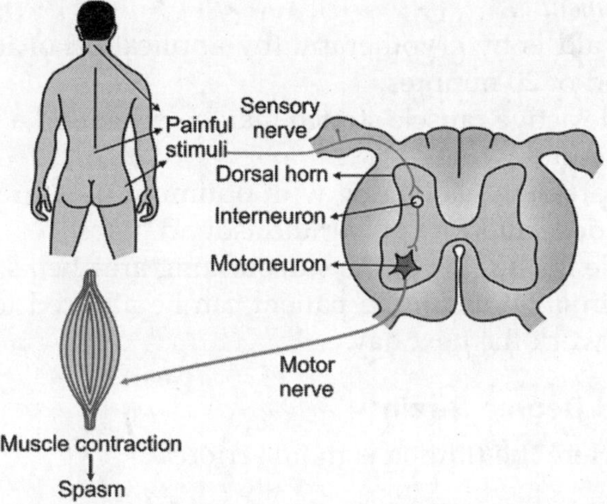

Fig. 2.4: Induction of prolonged muscle contractions (spasm) by peripheral nociceptive stimuli

Clinical Features

- Localized pain and tenderness.
- Pain and spasm prevents muscle stretching.
- Function is not impaired largely.
- Tenderness over the affected muscles.

All the above features are shown in Fig. 2.5.

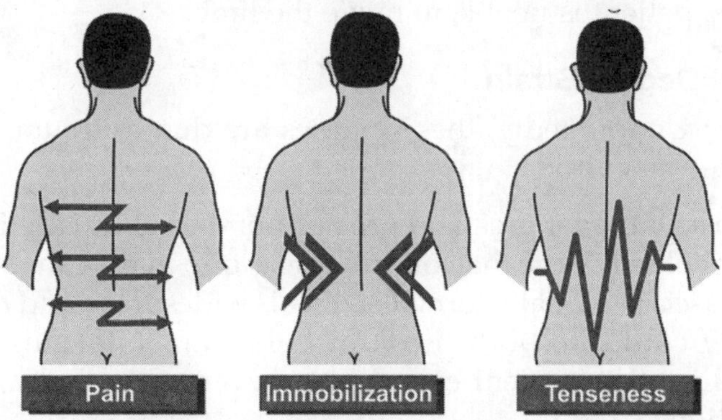

Fig. 2.5: Main symptoms of continuous muscle contractions (muscle spasms) in locomotors system: Pain, immobilization and tenseness-tenderness of muscles

Management

- First aid is by cryotherapy (by application of ice) for a period of 20 minutes.
- Gentle active muscle stretch may be permitted after 20 to 60 minutes.
- Compression bandaging with optimum pressure.
- Low dose and low power ultrasound helps.
- Gentle massaging of the surrounding area helps.
- If pain is minimal, the patient can be allowed to do the light work the next day.

Second Degree Strain

Cause: Here the trauma is more serious.

Pathology

- Greater number of muscle fibers is torn.
- There is bleeding.
- The fascia is still intact.
- Hematoma is still localized.

Symptoms

- Pain is more severe.
- Tenderness is severe.
- Severe muscle spasm.
- The patient is unable to move the limb.

Third Degree Strain

Cause: Undoubtedly, these injuries are due to trauma of a greater magnitude.

Pathology: Larger area and greater number of muscle fibers are involved. More than one muscle group may be involved. The fascia is partially torn. Bleeding is widespread and more. There could be both intramuscular and intermuscular bleeding. The patient experiences severe pain and loss of function.

Symptoms: Here all the above symptoms are of greater intensity.

Treatment in Grade II and III Strains

For first 24 hours

- Immediate application of ice.
- Compression bandage.
- Limb elevation.
- Limb immobilized in splints.
- Isometrics to the muscles, which are immobilized.
- Active exercises to the unaffected joints.
- Pulsed electromagnetic field therapy (PEMF) is known to help.
- No active movements to the affected muscles.

During the next 24 to 48 hours

- The pressure bandage is removed and active muscle exercises are begun.
- Stretching within the limits of pain is commenced.
- Thermotherapy: Ultrasound, short wave diathermy and TENS help to relieve pain.
- Slow rhythmic massaging helps relieve the muscle spasm.
- Nonweight bearing on crutches is slowly started.
- Rest of the measures is the same as above.

Between 48 and 72 hours

Apart from all the measures mentioned so far, the additional measures during this phase include:

- More vigorous active movements are encouraged.
- Deep transverse friction massage is added.
- Partial weight bearing can be permitted.

After 72 hours

- All the above measures are pursued in a more vigorous manner.
- Pressure bandage is totally removed.
- Progressive resisted exercises using the Fowler technique by taking out 10 to 12 repetition maximum (RM), is practiced.
- Full weight bearing should be permitted in injuries of the lower limbs.

- After full movement is regained, the patient is allowed to walk and jog.
- Full functional activity should be regained by 4 to 6 weeks. The various drugs used in the treatment of muscle strain to relieve pain and muscle stiffness is depicted in Table 2.1.

Table 2.1: Treatment of muscle strain by conservative methods in a nutshell

Systemic Therapy
Analgesic anti-inflammatory drugs
Antipyretic analgesics
Nonsteroidal anti-inflammatory drugs
Narcotic analgesics
Muscle relaxants
At muscular level
At neuromuscular level
At spinal level
At supraspinal level
Psychotropic drugs
Antidepressants
Neuroleptics
Minor tranquillizers
Others
Calcitonin
Beta-blockers
Local Therapy
Local anesthetics
Steroids
Transdermal application of analgesic anti-inflammatory drugs (ointments)

Grade Four Strain

Cause: This is usually caused by severe trauma.

Pathology

- Complete tear of the muscle (Figs 2.6A and B).
- The fascia is torn.
- Considerable bleeding which is intramuscular and diffuse.
- Gross swelling is present.

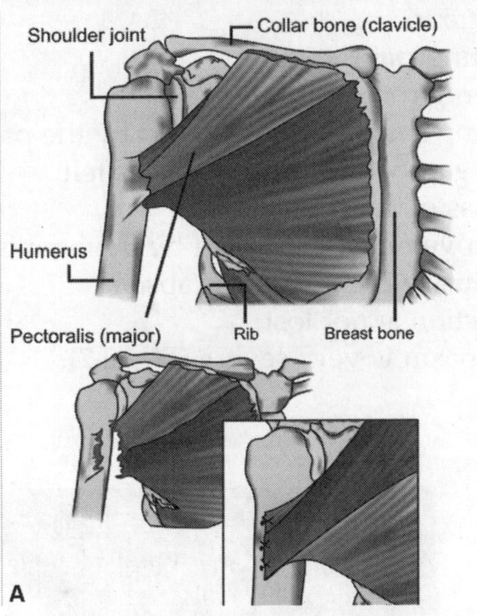

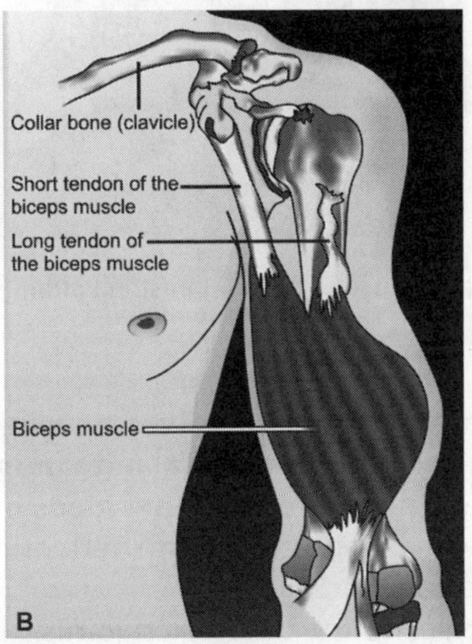

Figs 2.6A and B: Muscle ruptures that are common: (A) Rupture of pectoralis major muscle, and (B) Rupture of biceps tendon

Clinical Features

- Excruciating pain.
- Severe tenderness is present.
- A snapping sound may be heard by the patient.
- Palpable gap between the muscles felt.
- Severe loss of function.
- Active movements produced by the agonist are absent.
- Active muscle contraction is absent.
- Joint function is not lost.
- Muscle spasm is very severe (Fig. 2.7).

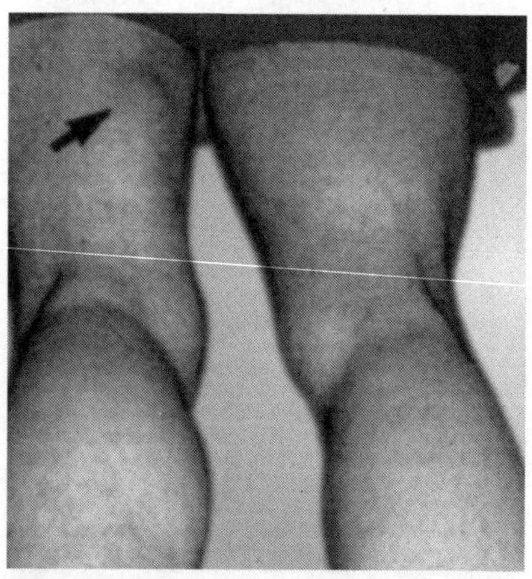

Fig. 2.7: Grade IV muscle strain (Hamstring strain) (Clinical photo)

Treatment

- Surgery is advised. This involves opening the ruptured site, evacuating the hematoma and suturing the fascial sheath. Direct muscle repair is avoided.
- Compression bandage is applied and the limb is immobilized for 2 to 3 weeks.
- Active exercises to the unaffected joints.
- Slow rhythmic isometric exercises to the affected muscles.
- Non-weight bearing after 48 hours.

- The use of low frequency current (faradism) to obtain passive contraction is very useful.
- Deep heating modalities like ultrasound, etc. help.
- Rest of the measures is same as for Grade II/III injuries.

Note: Mild muscle strain is also called by lay public as muscle pull.

INJURIES TO THE JOINTS

During an injury to a joint, three things could happen:

- Injury to the ligaments only
- Injury to the synovium
- Both (according to Bass, 1969).

Ligament Injury

A ligament injury is called "Sprain". Depending on the severity, it could be mild (Grade I), moderate (Grade II) or severe (Grade III).

Anatomy

Ligaments are made of fibrous tissues, which are arranged longitudinally. They are tough and elastic. Their vascularity is poor and heals always by scar tissue due to lack of special cells.

Functions

Ligaments serve the following functions:

Support: By reinforcing the capsule, they provide support to the joint.

Stability: By holding the bony ends together, it provides stability.

Protection: The strength of the ligaments offers protection to the joints along with the muscles.

Problems of Healing

- Poor vascularity delays the healing.
- Repair is by scar tissue.

- Inadequate period of immobilization results in healing with tissue that is more fibrous. This will result in excessive laxity making the joint unstable.
- Intermittent stretching strengthens the ligament while continuous stretch leads to adhesions due to periosteal irritation.

Types of Sprain (Fig. 2.8)

Grade I (Minor)

- Slight pain and tenderness at the site of injury.
- Slight swelling and loss of function.
- Stretch test will be positive clinching the diagnosis.

Treatment

First day

- Cryotherapy to alleviate pain.
- Pressure bandage—to prevent swelling.
- Limb elevation—to prevent swelling.
- Active movements of the unaffected joints.

Second day onwards

- Add thermotherapy, stop ice therapy.
- Begin isometric exercises to the affected muscles.

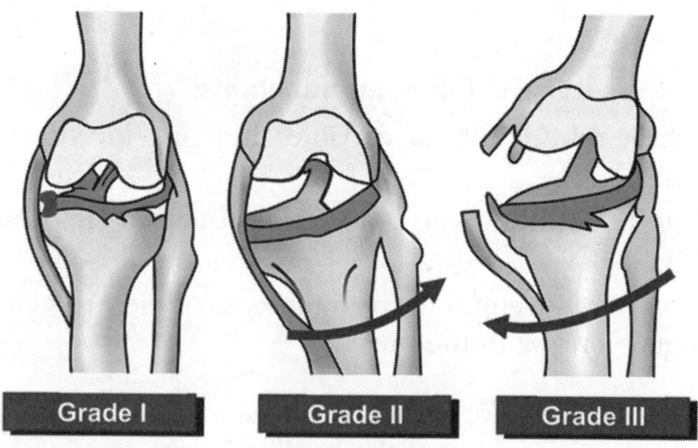

Fig. 2.8: Sprain of medial collateral ligament of the knee

- Weight bearing may be permitted.
- Rest of the measures is same as mentioned above.

Grade II (Severe)

- More force results in this injury.
- The ligament may be partially torn or detached from the attachment.
- Swelling is more severe.
- Pain and tenderness are also more acute.
- Movement is grossly restricted.
- Weight bearing is difficult.
- Function is severely affected.

Treatment

- Cryotherapy.
- Compression bandaging or kneecap and braces (Fig. 2.9).
- Elevation.
- Rest of the measures same as in Grade I.

Grade III (Complete rupture)

- Severe violence.
- Gross swelling.
- Pain and tenderness is quite severe.

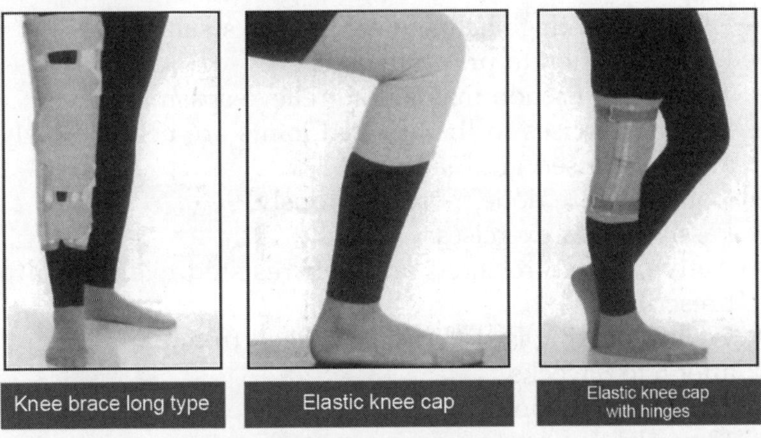

Fig. 2.9: Various elastic knee braces to support the knee joint

- Joint is unstable.
- The patient is unable to bear weight.
- Severe loss of function.

Treatment

- *Conservative*
  - Immediate application of ice.
  - Compression bandaging.
  - Foot end elevation.
  - Isometric exercises to the affected limbs.
  - Active exercises to affected joints.
  - POP cast for 6 to 8 weeks if ligament tear does not cause displacement.
- *Surgical*
  - If the ligament is torn and displaced, it needs surgical repair and immobilization with a POP cast for 6 to 8 weeks.
  - Isometric exercises are started after one week.
  - Non-weight-bearing for 3 to 4 weeks.

After Removal of the POP Cast

- *Thermotherapy:* Ultrasound, TENS or SWD helps to relieve pain.
- Pressure bandage helps to control the swelling.
- Limb elevation to prevent edema.
- Transverse friction massage to relieve spasm.
- Active exercises to the affected joints are begun slowly and progressed gradually.
- Isometrics are done more vigorously.
- Passive ROM exercises.
- Active, active-resisted and self-resisted exercises are prescribed.
- Weight-bearing is slowly encouraged from partial to full after 6 to 8 weeks.
- The patient should be functionally independent by 8 to 12 weeks.

Injury to the Synovium

Relevant Anatomy

Synovium is a lining covering the capsule of the joint, tendon sheaths, etc. It has a rich blood and nerve supply. It is present throughout the body.

Functions

Synovium produces synovial fluid, which serves the following functions:
- Facilitates frictionless, smooth joint movements.
- Helps in the nourishment of cartilages.

Causes

Inflammation of synovium is called *synovitis*. It could be due to trauma, arthritis, chondromalacia, rheumatoid arthritis, TB, hemophilia, etc.

Types

- Acute—due to trauma.
- Chronic—due to diseases like TB, rheumatoid arthritis, trauma, etc.

Clinical Features in Synovitis

- Swelling of the joint (develops slowly say within 2 to 24 hours).
- The joint is hot and red.
- Pain is present over the injured structure.
- Feeling of tension or pressure due to swelling.
- To accommodate the excess fluid, the joint will assume a flexion attitude (position of ease).
- Muscle atrophy will be quite significant.

In the Event of Synovial Rupture

- The patient feels sudden pain at the back of the knee while getting up from a chair, getting down the stairs, etc.
- The swelling may spread rapidly to the calf muscles. Homan's sign will be positive.

Treatment

Aim: To prevent muscle atrophy and joint contractures by a graduated exercise regimen.

Methods

During first 24 hours

- Ice therapy.
- Compression bandage.
- Limb elevation.
- Isometric contraction of the affected limb muscles.
- Active movements of the ankle joint.
- Active movements of the unaffected joints.
- Splinting of the affected part.

After 48 hours

- Aspiration of the joint if swelling persists even after 48 hours. Aspiration of the knee should be done in major OT under full aseptic conditions by giving local anesthesia. The technique of knee aspiration is shown in Figs 2.10A to E.
- Sustained isometric contraction of the muscles.
- Small range gradual active movements with adequate support should now be begun.
- Partial weight bearing may be allowed.
- Gradually progressive resistive exercises should be started to achieve full function.

Note: Hemarthrosis vs. synovitis
In hemarthrosis:
- The swelling is rapid in onset (< 2 hours).
- Swelling is more generalized.
- Pain on extreme movements.
- Joint instability may be present in cases of complete rupture.

Chronic Synovitis

This is due to various diseases affecting the synovium usually of more than three weeks' duration.

Tuberculosis of the joints, rheumatoid arthritis, etc. are some of the examples.

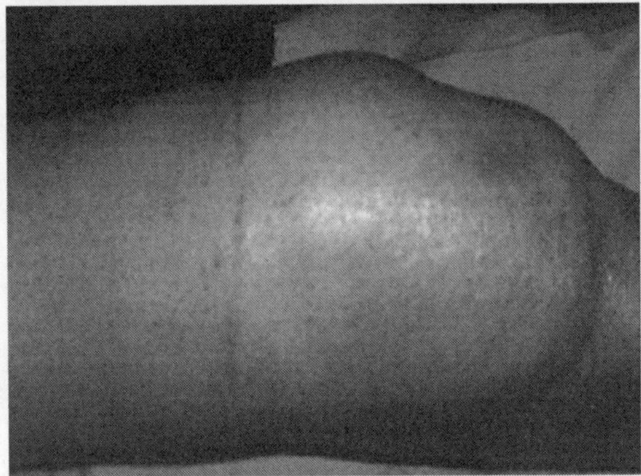

Fig. 2.10A: Gross swelling of the knee (Clinical photo)

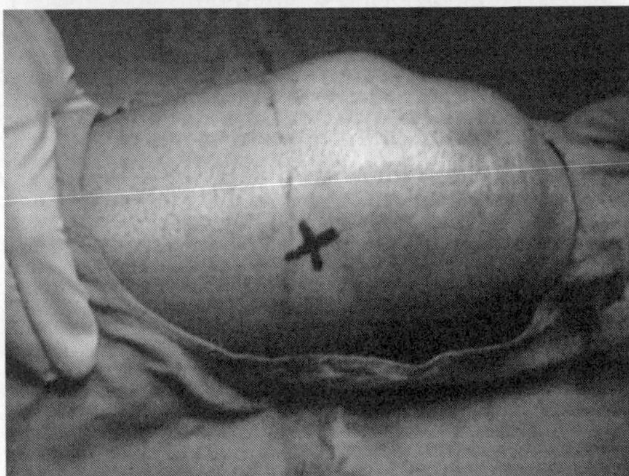

Fig. 2.10B: Mark the point of aspiration

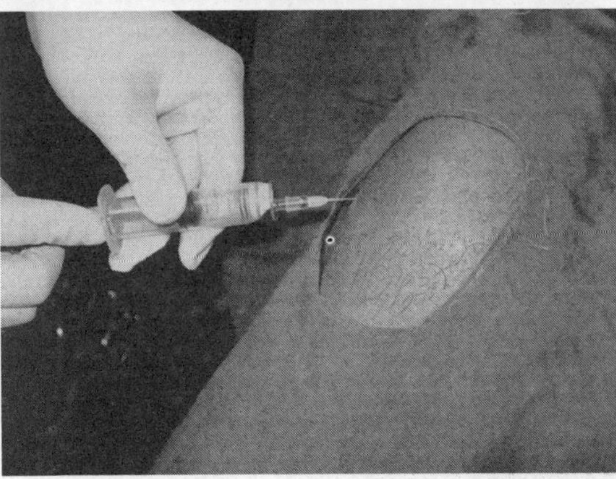

Fig. 2.10C: Part prepared and draped, local anesthesia given

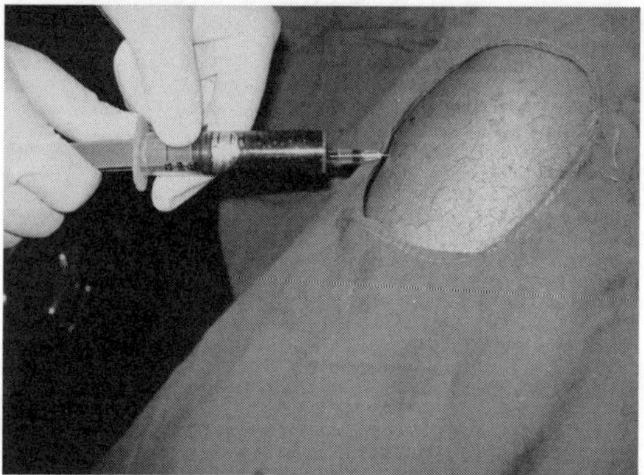

Fig. 2.10D: Thick blood being drained out

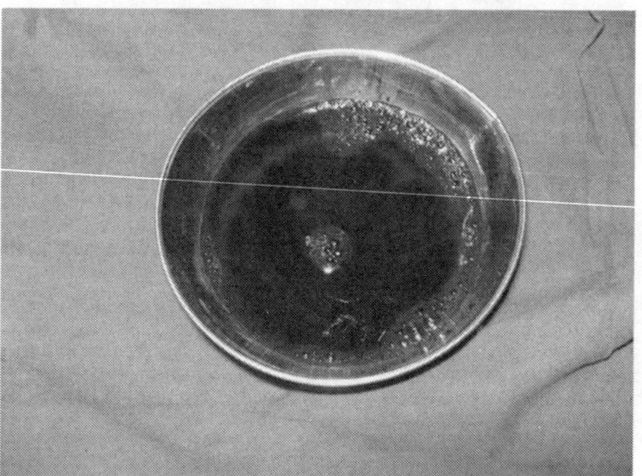

Fig. 2.10E: Frank thick blood devoid of fat globules

Problems of chronic synovitis

- Firm swelling.
- Muscle atrophy may be gross.
- Joint stiffness may be considerable.
- Lax ligaments create instability.
- Mild pain unlike acute synovitis.

Treatment

- Resistive exercises to the affected limbs.
- Isometric exercises to the affected parts.

- Passive ROM exercises to over come joint stiffness.
- Proper gait training.
- Ultrasound, TENS, SWD and other heat modalities to overcome pain and spasm.

Injury to the Bursa

Bursa is thin membranous sac lined with synovial membrane situated at the ends or certain important locations of the bones where tendons, etc. pass over them (Fig. 2.11).

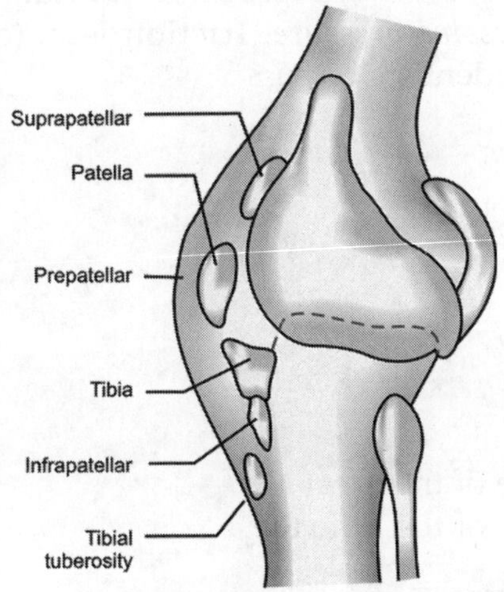

Fig. 2.11: Knee joint has many bursae around it

Functions

- To prevent friction between two structures like tendons and bones that is liable to be rubbed against each other.
- To prevent wear and tear of muscles and tendons.
- To protect the structures from pressure and injury.

Types

True bursa: They are normally present in the body at certain important situations like beneath the acromion, elbow, knee, heel, etc.

False bursa: They are also called as adventitious bursa. They develop due to external trauma, pressure, etc.

Causes

The causes of bursitis are as follows:
- *Trauma* may be due to a single blow or repetitive trauma.
- *Infection* acute or chronic (e.g. TB).
- *Metabolic disorders,* e.g. gout.
- *Abnormal external pressures,* etc. (e.g. hip ischial tuberosity).
- *Inflammatory disorders,* e.g. rheumatoid arthritis.
- *Unaccustomed activity,* exercise or ill-fitting shoes, etc.
- *Due to excessive pressure,* friction, etc. (e.g. olecranon bursitis, student's elbow).

Common Sites

Upper Limbs

a. Subacromion
b. Olecranon

Lower Limbs

a. Prepatellar
b. Tendo-Achilles
c. Medial side of the great toe
d. Lateral side of the little toe.

Clinical Features

- Pain, more so if it ruptures.
- Swelling is tender and hot.
- Movements of the joint may be painful.
- Tenderness may be present.
- Limp due to glutei bursitis, etc.

Treatment

In bursitis due to friction

- Rest to the part.
- Thermotherapy: US, SWD, TENS, etc.
- Cryotherapy in initial stages (first 24 to 48 hours).

- Restricted weight bearing.
- Isometric exercises to the affected part.
- Muscle strengthening exercises.
- Joint mobilization if there is restriction.
- Injection of hydrocortisone in intractable cases.
- Excision of the bursa, if chronic and troublesome.

Infective bursitis

- Appropriate antibiotics
- Rest of the measures is same as above.

Chronic cases

- Appropriate supports like felt pad, footwear modifications, etc.
- Avoiding repeated frictional movements (E.g. shoulder abduction in subdeltoid bursa).
- Relaxed passive movements to avoid friction.
- Active limited ROM exercises with strong isometrics.
- Progressive resistive exercises.
- Deep heating like US, SWD, TENS, etc.
- Deep friction massage.
- Active exercises to the unaffected joints.
- Isometrics with limb in elevation helps considerably.

Tenosynovitis

This is due to inflammation of the synovial lining of the tendon sheath. The fibrous sheath is, however, not affected.

Types

Irritative: Due to abnormal or excessive friction. There is pain and crepitus on palpation. The movements are not affected and there are no adhesions. There is watery effusion due to sheath inflammation.

Infective: May be due to acute pyogenic infection or chronic infection like TB, etc.

Treatment

Irritative

- Rest to the part by appropriate splints.
- Avoid movements at the joints.
- Bandaging or POP cast.
- Thermotherapy, US, SWD or TENS.
- Deep friction massage.
- Difficult cases, hydrocortisone injection.
- Intractable cases, surgical excision.
- Shoe modifications, etc.

Infective

- Appropriate antibiotics.
- Immobilization for 2 to 3 months.
- Rest of the measures is the same as mentioned above.

Tenovaginitis

Unlike in tenosynovitis, here the fibrous sheath and not the synovial sheath of the tendon are affected. Though patient may complain of pain, crepitus is conspicuous by its absence, e.g. de Quervain's disease (Fig. 2.12).

Though the exact cause is unknown (Adams 1981), Cyrius (1978) says it may be due to repeated strains. Infection is not known to cause this problem.

Treatment

This is similar to tenosynovitis.

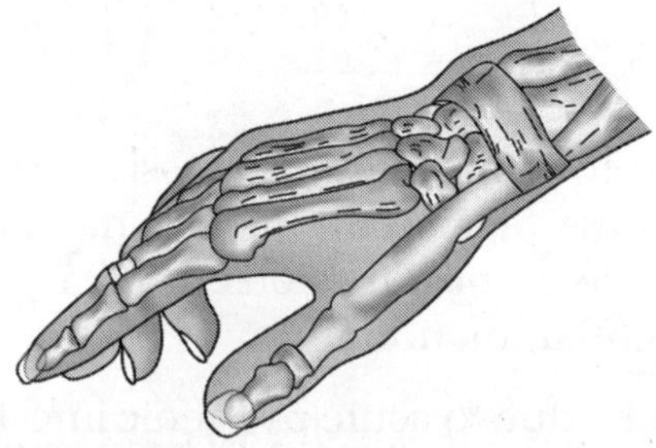

Fig. 2.12: de Quervain's disease: an example of tenovaginitis

SPECIAL TYPES OF MUSCLE INJURIES

- **Bruise or contusion:** It is nothing but the Grade I muscle strain. This has already been discussed and is called a superficial hematoma.
- **Hematomas:** These are deep in nature and two types are described:

Intramuscular Hematoma

- Here blood is contained within the muscle and is bound by an intact muscle sheath.
- Following an injury, bleeding occurs and stops within two hours.
- There is localized swelling.
- If there is further trauma, more bleeding may occur.

Intermuscular Hematoma

- Here the sheath of the muscle is torn resulting in extravasations of blood between the muscle and fascial planes.
- The hematoma is more diffuse.
- Bleeding will be more as the tension does not build-up to stop it.
- Due to gravity, it tracks down and may cause discoloration beneath the skin.
- For the first 48 hours it is difficult to differentiate between the above hematomas (Fig. 2.13).

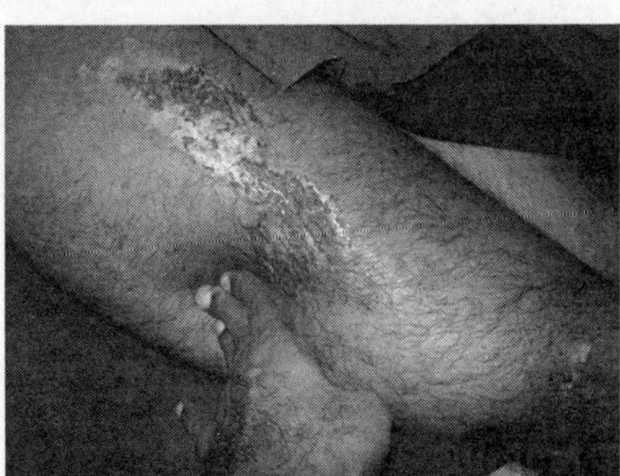

Fig. 2.13: Hematoma of the thigh (Clinical photo)

Quick facts

Features of intermuscular hematomas
- Moderate pain
- Swelling reduces drastically by 48 to 72 hours
- Muscle contraction is regained first
- Due to tracking swelling may be seen at a distance away from the site of injury.

Treatment

Aim is to prevent further bleeding.

Methods

- Rest to the part
- Immobilize the affected part with splint
- Cryotherapy to relieve pain and spasm
- Pressure bandage to control the swelling
- Limb elevation to prevent edema.

Note: In hematomas there is no loss of function. If there is loss of function then it may be a Grade II/III muscle strain.

IMPORTANT SOFT TISSUE PROBLEMS

Given below is a list of important soft tissue problems in orthopedics. Please refer the appropriate sections for details.

Upper Limb

Shoulder

- Rotator cuff injuries.
- Supraspinatus tendonitis.
- Infraspinatus tendonitis
- Subscapularis tendonitis
- Adhesive capsulitis.
- Tendonitis of the long head of biceps.

Elbow

- Tennis elbow.
- Golfer's elbow.
- Student's or miner's elbow.

Wrist

- Ganglion.
- de Quervain's disease.
- Dupuytren's contracture.
- Trigger finger.
- Carpal tunnel syndrome.
- Mallet finger.

Lower Limbs

Hip and Pelvis

- Piriformis syndrome
- Iliotibial tract syndrome
- Glutei bursitis
- Trochanteric bursitis.

Knee and Leg

- Bursa around the knee.
- Collateral ligament injury.
- Cruciate ligament injury.
- Meniscal injury.
- Quadriceps strain.
- Hamstrings strain
- Calf muscle strain
- Patellar tendonitis
- Plica syndrome.

Ankle and Foot

- Ankle sprain.
- Plantar fasciitis.
- Calcaneal spur.
- Morton's neuroma.
- Tendo-Achilles injuries.
- Tarsal tunnel syndrome.

Tendons and Nerves

- Injuries of flexor and extensor tendons of the hand.
- Injuries to the nerves please refer to chapter "Peripheral Nerve Injuries" in the book on Spinal Injuries.

3 Upper Limb Injuries in Sports

Given below is a list of important soft tissue problems of the upper limb in orthopedics. Please refer the appropriate sections for Details.

Upper Limb

Shoulder

- Rotator cuff injuries
- Supraspinatus tendonitis
- Infraspinatus tendonitis
- Subscapularis tendonitis
- Tendonitis of the long head of biceps.

Elbow

- Tennis elbow
- Golfer's elbow

Wrist and Hand

- de Quervain's disease
- Carpal tunnel syndrome
- Mallet finger

Now let us analyse each of these sports injuries in detail.

Note: Rotator cuff comprises supraspinatus, infraspinatus, subscapularis and teres minor (Mnemonic SITS).

UPPER LIMB SPORTS INJURIES

SHOULDER INJURIES

ROTATOR CUFF LESIONS

This includes both rotator cuff tears and impingement syndrome. Fine adjustments of the humeral head within the glenoid is achieved by coordinated activity of four interrelated muscles (Fig. 3.1) arising from the scapula and is called *rotator cuff.*

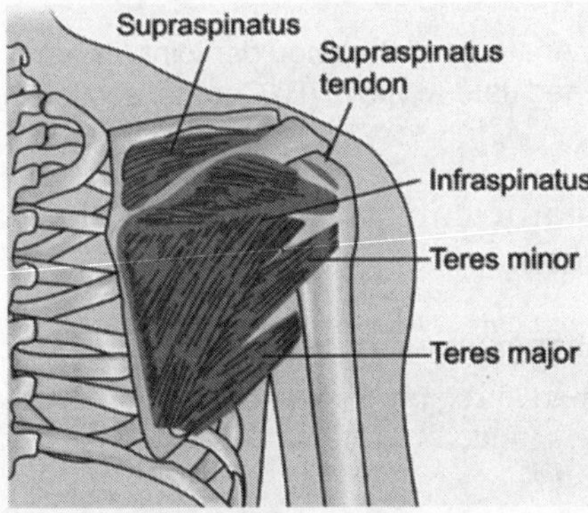

Fig. 3.1: Muscles of the rotator cuff

Role of Rotator Cuffs

In the movement of abduction, supraspinatus steadies the head from above, infraspinatus depresses the head, and subscapularis steadies the head in front paralleling the action of the infraspinatus. *This combined action allows the deltoid muscle to swing up the arm from a steady fulcrum irrespective of the position of the scapula* (Figs 3.2A and B).

Impingement Syndrome

It is a problem, which is commonly associated with supraspinatus tendon. Other causes like bicipital tendonitis, and intraspinatus tendonitis, subacromial bursitis, etc. may

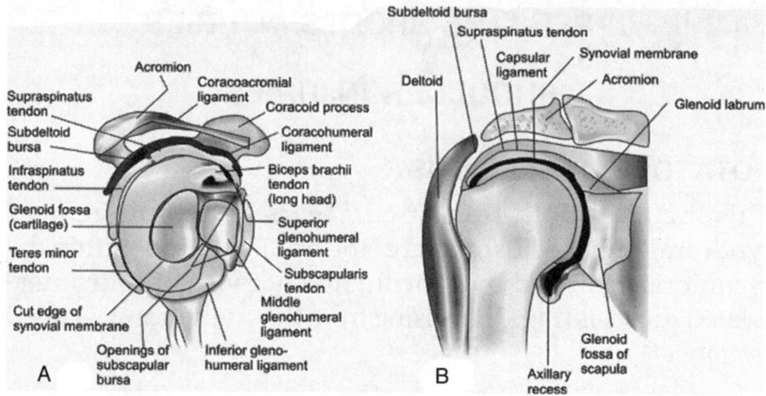

Figs 3.2A and B: Anatomy of the shoulder joint (internal structures): (A) Shoulder joint opened (lateral view), (B) Coronal section through shoulder joint

give rise to rotator cuff problems, but they are not that common (see box).

Causes of impingement syndrome

- Complete or partial rupture of rotator cuff.
- Supraspinatus tendonitis.
- Calcific deposits.
- Subacromial bursitis.
- Subdeltoid bursitis.
- Periarthritis.
- Bicipital tenosynovitis.
- Fracture greater trochanter.

SUPRASPINATUS TENDINITIS

Among the various causes mentioned above, supraspinatus tendinitis is the one that is commonly encountered and this gives rise to the *impingement syndrome.* Impingement occurs beneath the coracoacromial arch. The most vulnerable structures for impingement between the undersurface of the acromion and the head of the humerus are the greater tuberosity, the overlying supraspinatus tendon (Fig. 3.3) and the long head of biceps. The major site of compression is anterior to the angle of the acromion. Hence, the proper term is *anterior impingement syndrome* or painful arc syndrome (Fig. 3.4).

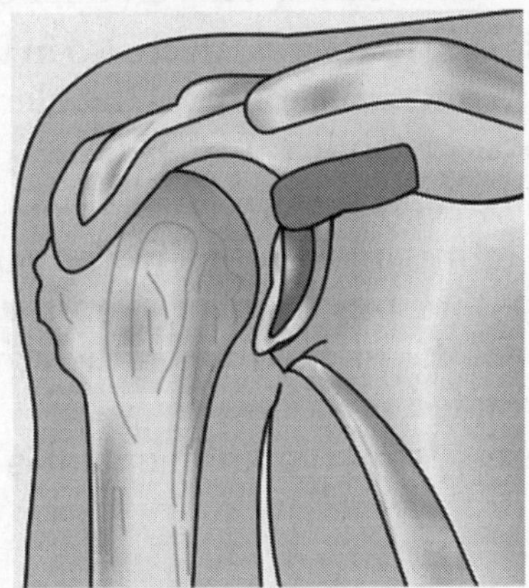

Fig. 3.3: Supraspinatus tear

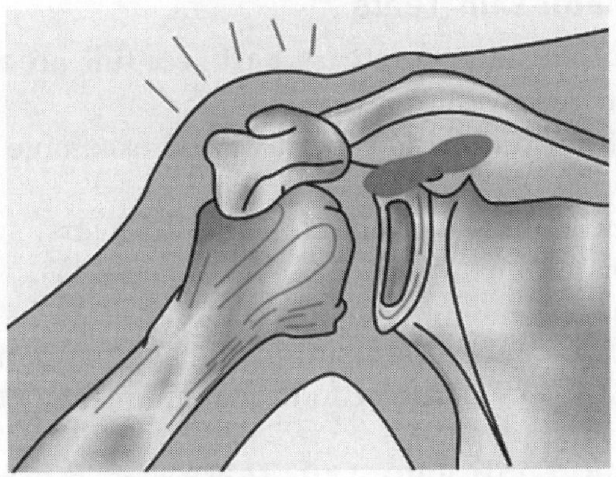

Fig. 3.4: Anterior impingement syndrome

Neer's stages of impingement syndrome

- Edema stage.
- Tendinitis and fibrositis.
- Rotator cuff tears and rupture of biceps tendon.
- Bone changes.

Types of Impingement Syndrome

Primary: Here impingement occurs beneath the coracoacromial arch and is due to subacromial overloading.

Secondary: This is due to relative decrease in the subacromial arch and is due to microinstability of the glenohumeral joint or scapulothoracic instability.

Posterior (Internal): Seen in overhead athletes like throwers, swimmers and tennis players. Here the supra and infraspinatus tendons are pinched between the posterior and superior aspects of the glenoid when the arm is in elevated and externally rotated position.

Among the three, primary impingement is more common.

ROTATOR CUFF TEARS

Note: Incidence of rotator cuff tear, less than 70 years—30 percent; 71–80 years—60 percent; more than 89 years—70 percent.

About Rotator Cuff Tears

The causes for rotator cuff tears, partial or full, are as follows:

- Age > 40 years.
- Occupations requiring repetitive and excessive overhead movements.
- Overhead sports and athletes like throwers, swimmers, tennis players, etc.
- Degenerative etiology is the major cause.
- Dislocation of shoulder joint in 40–60 years of age.
- About 2/3rd cases are seen in male population.

Classification of Rotator Cuff Tears

(According to American Arthroscopic Orthopedics)

- Small tear (< 1 cm)
- Medium tear (1–3 cm)
- Large tears (3–5 cm).

Clinical Tests

Special shoulder tests that are helpful in diagnosing

rotational, cuff tears and the impingement syndrome, is the ***painful arc sign*** (it is 81% specific). There are innumerable other tests but is outside the scope of this book.

Interesting facts

Do you know the clinical facts leading to the diagnosis of RCL tear?

- Age > 40 years.
- Previous history of minor trauma.
- Degenerative changes on the X-rays.
- Various clinical tests.
  How accurate are these tests?
  There are 91 percent sensitive and 75 percent specific.
  Pearl: Clinical tests are ***more*** accurate and cost-effective than a battery of investigations in diagnosing an RCL.

Clinical Features

All patients with impingement syndrome have similar clinical features like pain, swelling, limitation of shoulder movements, muscle atrophy (supraspinatus and infraspinatus), and tenderness over the greater tuberosity, etc. The following grades are described in anterior impingement syndrome.

Grade I: This is common in young adults and athletes in the age group of 18–30 years. Due to over stress and repeated overhead activity, impingement occurs and supraspinatus is inflamed. The painful arc appears here (Fig. 3.5).

Grade II: This is seen in age group of 40–45 years and may be due to supraspinatus tendinitis or subacromial bursitis. The cause could be either overuse or degeneration and osteophyte formation.

Grade III: It is seen in patients over 45 years of age and may be due to occupational overuse, fall, and sudden increase in activity, atrophic degenerative changes in the cuff and rarely due to acute tear of the rotator cuff.

Investigations to Diagnose Rotator Cuff Lesions

X-rays of the shoulder: This helps to detect bony avulsions, spurs, calcific deposits, sclerotic areas, etc. (Figs 3.6A and B).

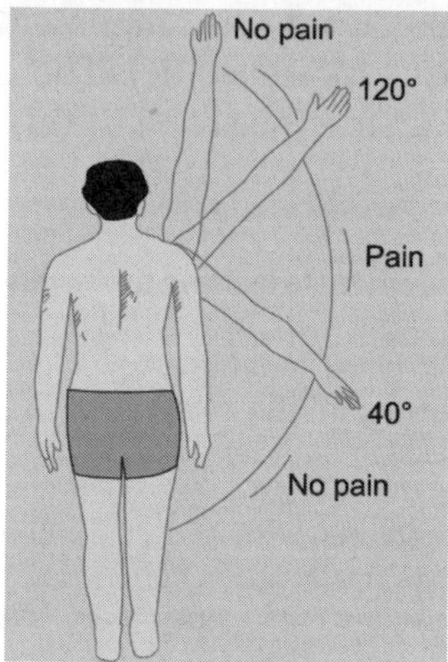

Fig. 3.5: Pain occurs in the impingement syndrome between 40° and 120° of shoulder abduction as it is in a position that the supraspinatus tendon is impinged against the undersurface of the acromion and head of the humerus. Rest of the movements are painless (painful are syndrome)

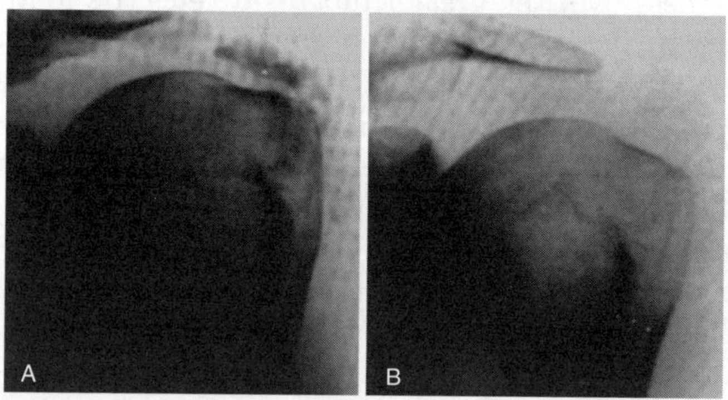

Figs 3.6A and B: Radiographs showing changes in the rotator cuff tears: (A) Calcific depositis, (B) Degenerative changes

Arthrogram: Single contrast arthrogram is considered as the gold standard in diagnosing rotator cuff tears.

Ultrasonography: This is highly reliable in diagnosing rotator cuff pathology with a sensitivity of 98 percent.

MRI: This is also very accurate (81%) but expensive.

Mystifying facts about X-ray changes in Rotator Cuff Lesions

- ↓ Subarachnoid space ↓ 6 mm.
- Anterior spurring of ACM joint.
- Humeral head degeneration.
- Sclerotic inferior acromion (eyebrow sign).
- Hooking of the acromion.

Management

Conservative Treatment

It consists of heat, massage, NSAIDs, local infiltration of hydrocortisone, subacromial steroid injections, exercises both active and passive, temporary immobilization, etc. *Ninety percent will recover with these measures.*

Surgical Treatment

Indications: Failure of conservative treatment for three months, if the patients are young and active, and if there is increasing loss of shoulder function, surgery is indicated.

Methods

- Arthroscopic repair in small and partial tears.
- Open methods in major tears.

Depending upon the etiological factors, the following surgical techniques are described: Excision of adhesions and manipulation of shoulder, excision of calcium deposits, repair of incomplete tear, acromioplasty, acromionectomy for more disabling pain with normal range of movements, direct suture for complete rupture of rotator cuff, rotation and transposition of flap, free graft, etc. Results are good in 85–90 percent.

Differential Diagnosis of Impingement Syndrome

- Frozen shoulder.
- Cervical spondylosis.
- ACM and shoulder joint arthritis.
- Bursitis.

- Snapping scapula.
- Suprascapular neuropathy.

FRACTURE CLAVICLE

The term clavicle (Fig. 3.7) is derived from the Latin root *Clavis* meaning *Key*. Clavicle is 'S' shaped and is linked to the music symbol 'clavicula', hence the name.

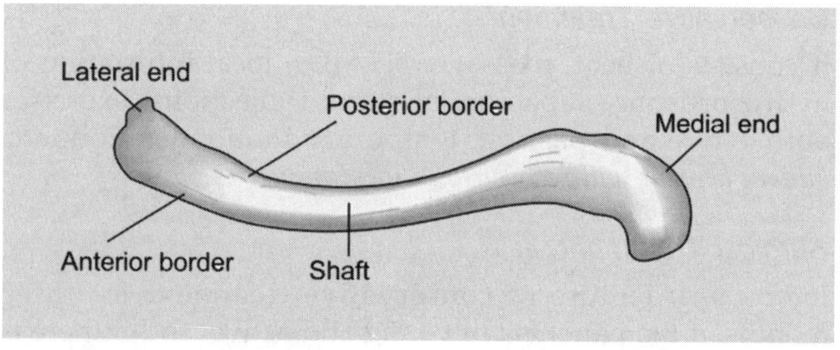

Fig. 3.7: Bony anatomy of the clavicle

Mechanism of Injury

Direct

Due to fall on the point of the shoulder. This is the most common mode of injury accounting for 91 percent of the cases.

Direct Trauma

Direct trauma over the clavicle due to RTA, direct injury, etc. accounts for 8 percent of the cases (Fig. 3.8).

Indirect fall on the outstretched hands accounts for 1 percent of the cases.

Sites of Fracture

- Eighty-five percent of the fracture clavicle occurs at the junction of middle and outer third (Fig. 3.9).
- One percent at the medial end of the clavicle (5%).

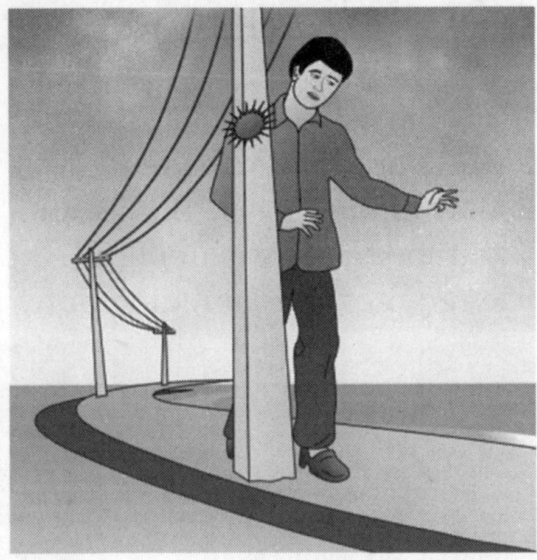

Fig. 3.8: Recklessness like this can break your clavicle bone due to direct injury

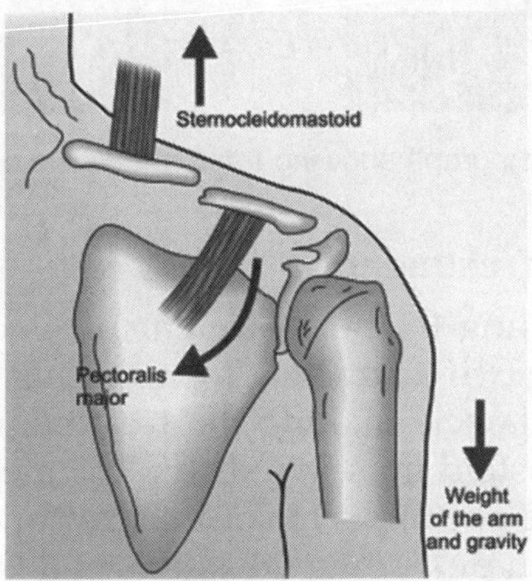

Fig. 3.9: Showing various displacing forces in fracture clavicle

- Lateral end fracture is uncommon (About 10%) (Distal 1/3rd).

Clinical Features

The patient presents with pain, swelling, deformity and inability to raise the shoulder. Rarely, the patient may present with pseudo-paralysis of the affected arm.

Radiographs

The following views are recommended:
- Routine AP view of the clavicle (Fig. 3.10).
- Lordotic view if the fracture is doubtful.
- Distal clavicle requires special radiography technique.

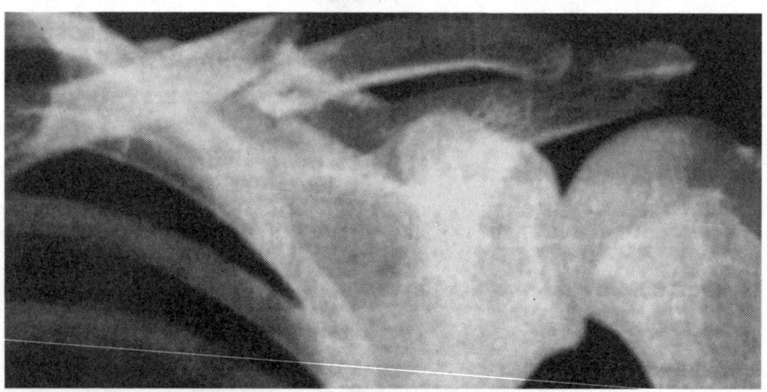

Fig. 3.10: Radiograph showing fracture clavicle of middle third

Principles of Treatment

Before proceeding to the treatment proper one needs to understand the two distracting forces acting on the fracture fragments in clavicle making the treatment difficult. The sternocleidomastoid muscle pulls up the medial end of the clavicle and the pectoralis major muscle and gravity acting through the arm pull down the lateral end (see Fig. 2.8).

To counter the above two detrimental forces, the shoulder should be braced up and back and the arm should be supported while treating fracture clavicle.

Conservative Methods

This is the treatment of choice in fracture clavicle and consists of the following methods:

Cuff and collar sling for undisplaced fractures (Fig. 3.11A).

Strapping of the fracture site after reduction of the fracture by elevating the arm and bracing the shoulder upwards and backwards gives good results in both children and adults (Fig. 3.11B).

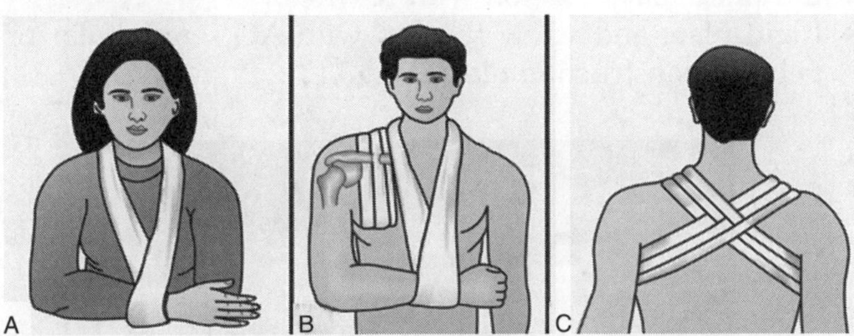

Figs 3.11A to C: Methods of conservative treatment of fractures clavicle: (A) Collar and cuff sling, (B) Strapping and sling suspension, and (C) Figure of '8' bandaging

Sabre method consists of rigid dressing over the fracture. This is no longer used.

Billington Yoke method uses a plaster of Paris over a well-padded figure of '8' dressing.

Figure of '8' is popularly used and it acts by retracting the shoulder girdle, minimizes the overlap and allows more anatomical healing. *It does not immobilize the fracture but acts by serving as a reminder to the patient to hold the shoulder up and back neutralizing the forces mentioned above. If they allow the shoulder to slump forward, then the support cuts into the anterior axilla and reminds them to hold the shoulders back* (Fig. 3.11C).

Treatment Plan

Newborn to perambulatory children: Treated symptomatically, bind arm to the chest.

Ambulatory stage (2–12 yr): Figure of '8' bandages, tightened after three days and later one week.

Twelve years to maturity: Commercially available figure of '8' harness.

Surgery is rarely indicated and consists of open reduction and rigid internal fixation.

Methods of Internal Fixation

- Intramedullary fixation with K-wires.
- Rigid plate and screw fixation with AO semitubular or pelvic reconstruction plate (Fig. 3.12).

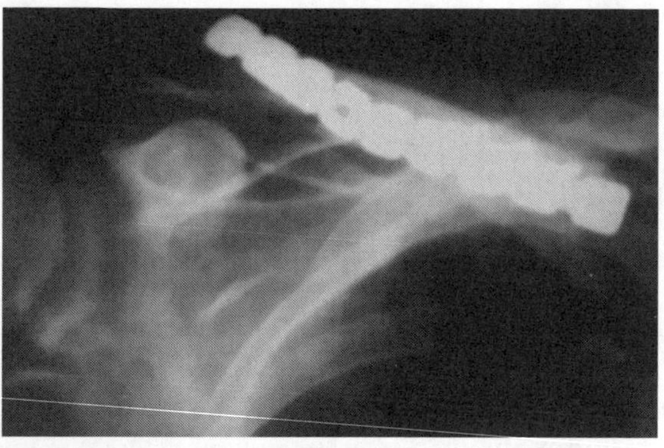

Fig. 3.12: Radiograph showing fracture clavicle plate fixation

Indications

Open fractures, injury to neurovascular bundle, if the fracture is threatening to penetrate the skin, nonunion, fracture near acromioclavicular joint, floating shoulder, soft tissue interposition and displaced epiphysis in children.

INJURIES OF THE ACROMIOCLAVICULAR JOINT

Acromioclavicular (ACM) joint is a diarthrodial joint with a fibrocartilaginous disk between the two bones (similar to a meniscus).

Mechanism of Injury

Direct force is the most common mechanism (Fig. 3.13) of injury as in RTA, assault, athletic events like the tackling, etc.

Indirect force is due to fall on the outstretched hands.

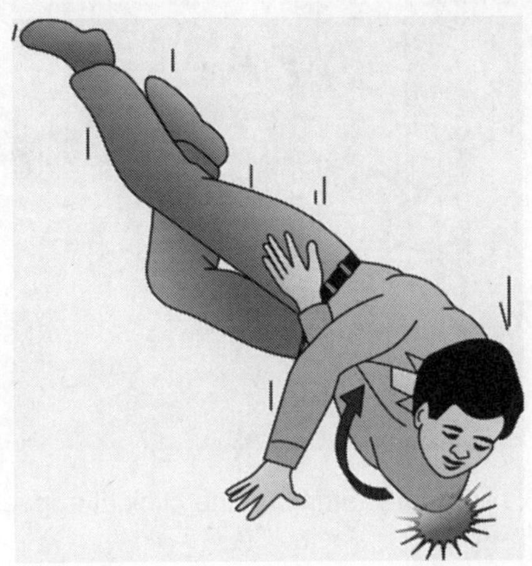

Fig. 3.13: Showing the most common mechanism of injury of ACM joint

Downward indirect force through the upper extremity is relatively rare.

Clinical Features

The patient complains of pain, swelling, and difficulty in raising the arm up. The patient supports the affected shoulder by holding the elbow with unaffected hand. On examination, there is tenderness and the lateral end of clavicle is prominently felt (Fig. 3.14).

Radiographs

The following views are required:

- AP view with 15° cephalic tilt to prevent overlap of the spine of scapula on routine AP views (Figs 3.15A and B).
- Lateral view—axillary view of the shoulder.
- Stress radiographs—to differentiate from type II and type III by suspending a weight of 10 to 15 lb around the wrist.

Management

Type I: Rest, ice bags, NSAIDs, etc.

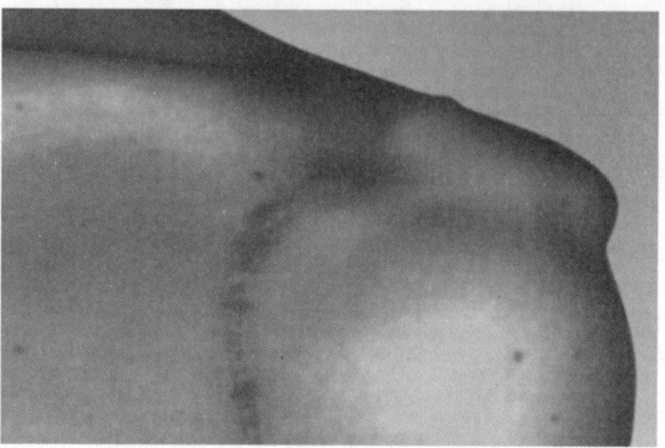

Fig. 3.14: ACM joint injury, the clinical appearance

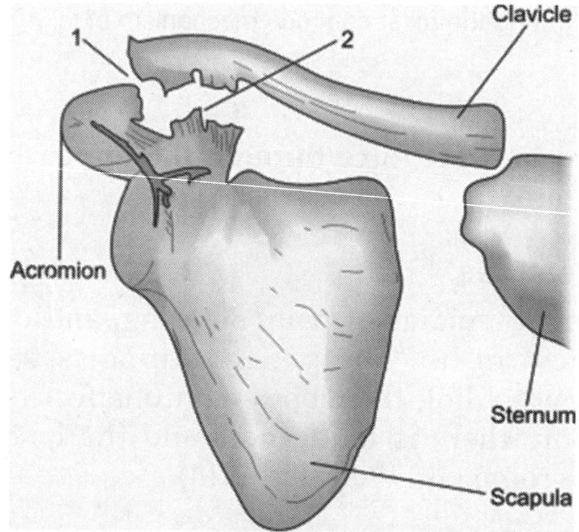

Fig. 3.15A: Acromioclavicular joint injury shows: (1) Ruptured acromioclavicular ligament (ACL), and (2) Ruptured coracoclavicular ligament (CCL)

Type II: Sling for 10 to 14 days, adhesive strapping, elastic strapping, cast or harness. Surgery is required for persisting pain.

Type III: Conservative methods like reduction and retention with sling and harness.

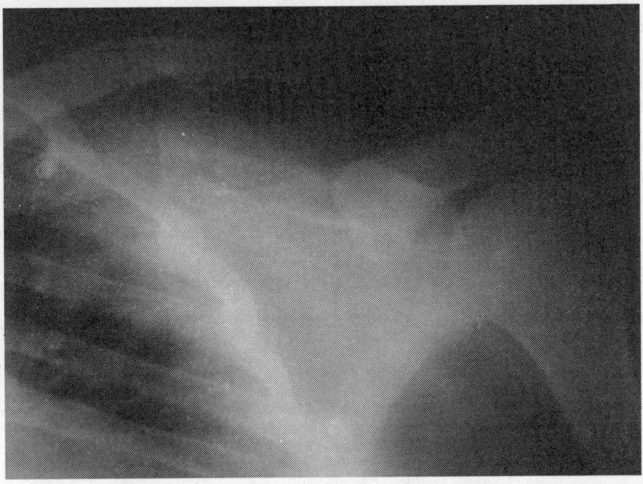

Fig. 3.15B: Radiograph showing ACM joint dislocation

Surgical methods include:
- Acromioclavicular repair.
- Coracoclavicular repair.
- Excision of distal end of clavicle for old symptomatic cases.
- Dynamic muscle transfer by transferring the coracoid process.

Types IV, V and VI: Require open reduction, internal fixation, repair and reconstruction.

Complications

- Associated fracture clavicle.
- Coracoclavicular ossification.
- Osteolysis of distal clavicle.
- Complications after surgery like infection, etc.
- Complications after non-operative treatment like joint stiffness, periarthritis, etc.

Delayed complications: These include:
- Step-like deformity.
- ACM joint arthritis.
- Pain during weightlifting.

INJURIES OF STERNOCLAVICULAR JOINT

Mechanism of Injury

This is the least commonly dislocated joint because of the strong ligaments.

Direct force rarely causes this injury. For example, collision of an athlete with another person or a post, etc.

Indirect force is the most common mode of injury. For example, loading the upper shoulder while someone lies on the sides (Fig. 3.16A).

Incidence is about three percent and is more common in young males.

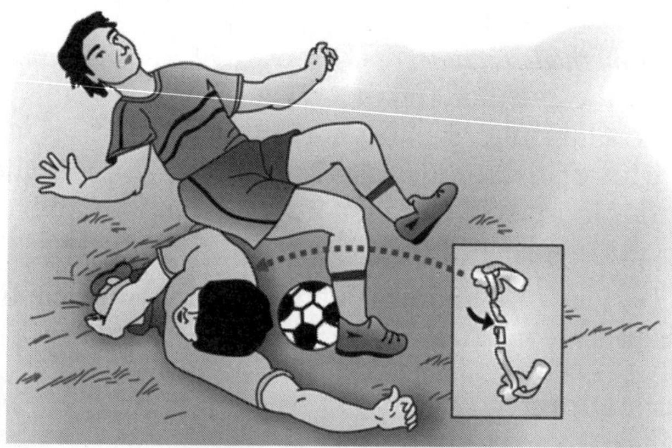

Fig. 3.16A: The most common mechanism of injury of the sternoclavicular joint

Causes

Road traffic accident (RTA) is responsible for 80 percent of the cases, sports-related injuries account for the remaining 20 percent.

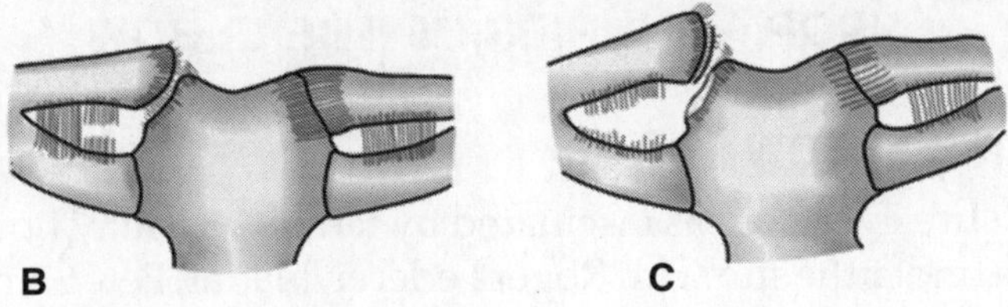

Figs 3.16B and C: Sternoclavicular joint injuries: (B) Partial separation, and (C) Total separation

Clinical Features

The patient complains of pain and swelling. Medial end of the clavicle is prominent in anterior dislocation. Affected shoulder is short. Lateral compression test is positive.

Radiographs

- AP view is often difficult to interpret.
- Special 90° cephalocaudal views—this helps to see the medial ends of both the clavicles (serendipity view).
- Tomograms are useful.
- CT scans and MRI help to study the position of clavicle with respect to sternum and soft tissues respectively.

Management

Mild sprain: The treatment consists of ice, sling, painkillers, etc.

Subluxation: The treatment methods are ice (first 12 hr), warmth (24–48 hr), clavicle strap, and figure of '8' and excision of medial end if pain persists.

Dislocation: The treatment of choice is closed reduction by firm digital pressure followed by figure of '8', clavicle strap, sling, etc. If it fails, open reduction and internal fixation using K-wire is done.

SPORT INJURIES OF THE ELBOW

TENNIS ELBOW

I am sure every one is fascinated by tennis. We may not get a place under the sun with Roger Federer, Nadaf, Pete Sampras, Leander Paes, Sania Mirza and others, but certainly, we may get an appointment with an orthopedic surgeon for a problem common in them, that too without playing tennis! Yes, the obvious reference is towards *tennis elbow.*

Note: Sachin Tendulkar should be credited for popularizing and creating lots of awareness and controversies about tennis elbow at least in our country.

History

It was first described from the *Writer's Cramps* by Range in 1873. It was Madris who called it as "tennis elbow" shortly thereafter.

Definition

Tennis elbow syndrome encompasses lateral, medial and posterior elbow symptoms. The one commonly encountered is the lateral tennis elbow which is known as the ***classical tennis elbow*** and is the *pain and tenderness on the lateral side of the elbow*, some well-defined and some vague, that results from repetitive stress.

Lateral Tennis Elbow

It is a lesion affecting the tendinous origin of common wrist extensors (Fig. 3.17). It is more common in men than women are and is believed to be a degenerative disorder.

Causes

Epicondylitis: This is due to single or multiple tears in the common extensor origin, periostitis, angiofibroblastic proliferation of extensor carpi radialis brevis (ECRB), etc.

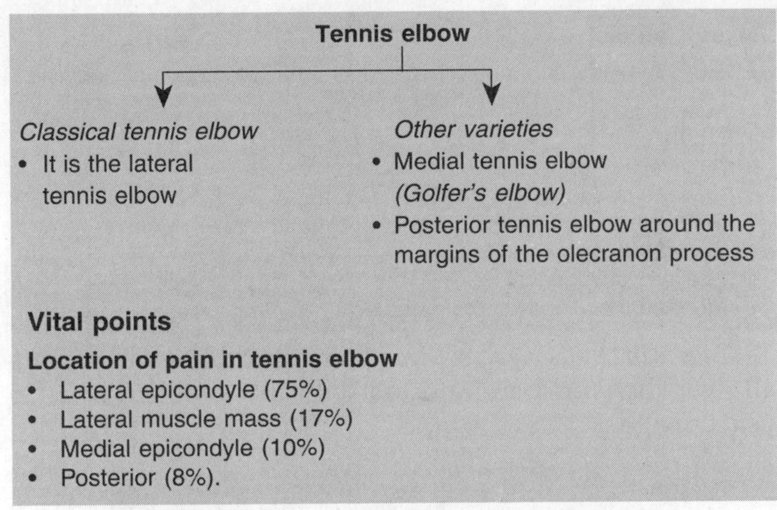

Tennis elbow

Classical tennis elbow
- It is the lateral tennis elbow

Other varieties
- Medial tennis elbow *(Golfer's elbow)*
- Posterior tennis elbow around the margins of the olecranon process

Vital points

Location of pain in tennis elbow
- Lateral epicondyle (75%)
- Lateral muscle mass (17%)
- Medial epicondyle (10%)
- Posterior (8%).

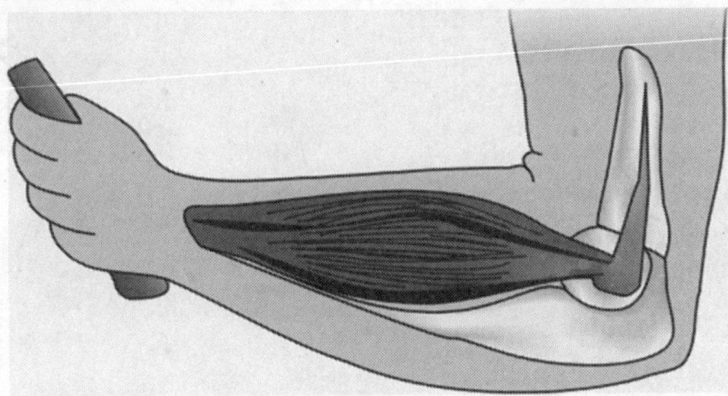

Fig. 3.17: Repetitive stress at common extensor origin in tennis players

Inflammation of adventitious bursa: Between the common extensor origin and radio humeral joint.

Calcified deposits: Within the common extensor tendon.

Painful annular ligament: It is due to hypertrophy of synovial fringe between the radial head and the capitulum's.

Pain of neurological origin, e.g. cervical spine affection, radial nerve entrapment.

Mystifying fact

ECRB is the most commonly involved structure in lateral epicondylitis.

Seen in

- All levels of tennis players.
- In world class players "SERVE" appears to be the cause.
- In less than world class players "backhand stroke".
- Seen in other sports also.
- May be occupational, etc.
- More common in the dominated arm.

Causes in tennis players: More than one-third tennis players all over the world are affected with this problem over 35 years of age.

- Novice.
- Playing several games per week.
- More than 35 years of age.
- Equal sex incidence.
- Backhand stroke (38%).
- Serve (25%).
- Forehand stroke (23%).
- Backhand volley (7%).
- Overhead smash (4%).
- Forehand volley (3%).

Contributing factors

- Little playing experience.
- Consistent missing of "*sweet spot*" while hitting.
- Poor stroke techniques: Use of arm instead of body.
- Poor power or flexibility.
- Heavy stiff racket, large handle size, too tight racket stringing.
- Heavy duty wet balls.
- Playing surface—balls bounce quicker off the cement court.

Did you know?

Though called tennis elbow, it is more common in non-tennis players (95%). Causes can be:

- Throwing sports
- Swimming
- Carpentry, plumbing, textile workers
- Housewives

However, up to 50 percent of tennis players suffer from this problem at some time in their sporting career.

Pathophysiology and Related Symptoms

Stage I: There is acute inflammation but no angioblastic invasion. *The patient complains of pain during activity.*

Stage II: This is the stage of chronic inflammation. There is some angioblastic invasion. *The patient complains of pain both during activity and at rest.*

Stage III: Chronic inflammation with extensive angioblastic invasion. *The patient complains pain at rest, night pains, and pain during daily activities.*

Etiology

Problems in tennis players: More than one-third tennis players all over the world are affected with this problem over 35 years of age are obviously due to faculty playing techniques.

Nontennis players: Ironically tennis elbow is more common in nontennis players. This unfortunate group is comprised of housewives, carpenters, miners, drill workers, etc. India's Cricketing Legend Sachin Tendulkar and SreeShanth have made tennis elbow very popular across the country and the world.

Indian housewives: This is the third largest group suffering from this condition. The household chores like washing, brooming, cooking, etc. require repeated extension of the elbow leading to the development of this condition.

Computer-related injuries: This is emerging as the recent epidemic among computer professionals across the globe due to repetitive stress while using laptops, mouse, etc.

Clinical Features

Patient complains of pain on the outer aspect of the elbow and has difficulty in gripping objects and lifting them. Sportspeople will have difficulty in extending the elbow. The following are some of the useful clinical tests.

Clinical Tests

Local tenderness on the outside of the elbow at the common extensor origin with aching pain in the back of the forearm (Fig. 3.18).

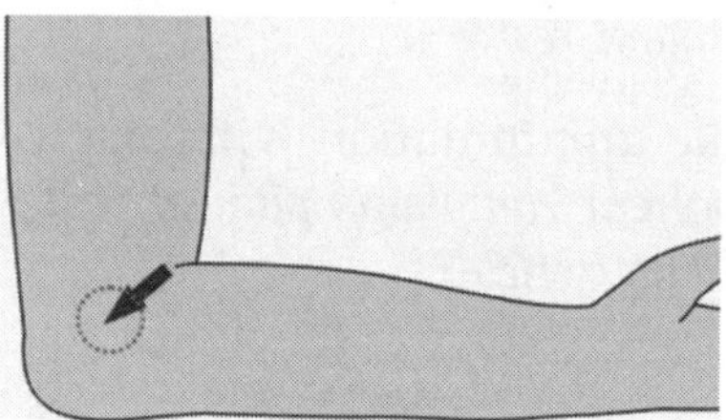

Fig. 3.18: Arrow showing site of tenderness in tennis elbow

Cozen's test: Painful resisted extension of the wrist with elbow in full extension elicits pain at the lateral elbow (Fig. 3.19).

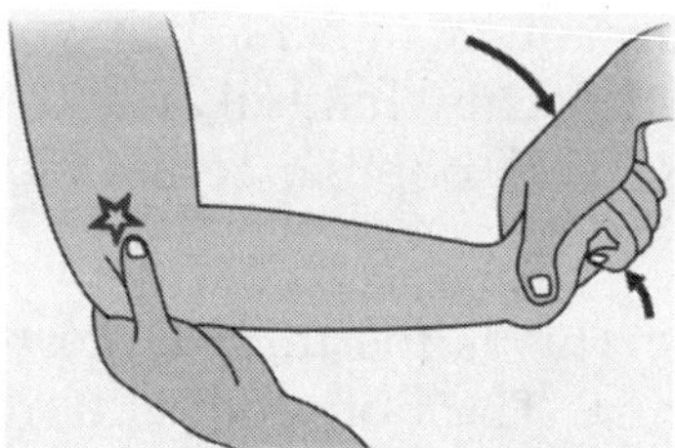

Fig. 3.19: Method of performing the Cozen's test

Elbow held in extension, passive wrist flexion and pronation produces pain.

Maudsley's test: Resisted extension of the middle finger (Remember the letter 'M') elicits pain at the lateral epicondyle due to disease in the extensor digitorum communis.

Radiograph for Tennis Elbow

The AP, lateral and radiocapitellar views are the recommended views. In most cases, it is normal. However, in 16 percent of the cases, a faint calcification along the lateral epicondyle can be detected.

Treatment

Conservative Management

It consists of rest and physiotherapy. In tennis players exercises, light racket, smaller grip, elbow strap, etc. are helpful (Fig. 3.20). Injection of local anesthetic and steroid are useful in 40 percent of cases.

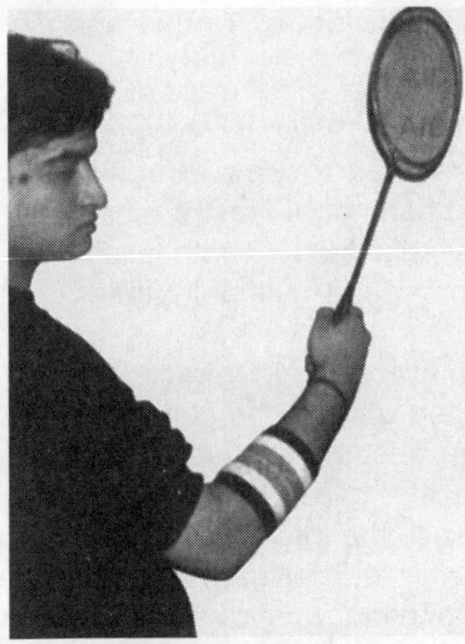

Fig. 3.20: Elbow supports to be used in tennis elbow

Mill's Maneuver

This is the final option before surgery. About 10 percent of the cases do not respond to conservative treatment. In them, a forceful extension of a fully flexed and pronated forearm after injection may be attempted.

Surgical Management

Indications

- Severe pain for 6 weeks at least.

- Marked and localized tenderness over lateral epicondyle.
- Failure to respond to restricted activity or immobilization for at least 2 weeks.

Surgical Methods

- Percutaneous release of epicondylar muscles.
- Bosworth technique of excision of the proximal portion of the annular ligament, release of the origin of the extensor muscles, excision of the bursa and excision of synovial fringes.

What is new in the treatment of Tennis and Golfer's elbow?

- *The use of extracorporeal shock wave therapy (ESWT):* About 2,000 shock waves of 0.04–0.12 nj/mm^2, three times at monthly intervals for 6 months are found to be effective in cases with failed conservative treatment for at least 6 months.
- *Arthroscopic release:* Of ECRB with failed conservative treatment for nearly 6 months. It is minimally invasive and helps in early rehabilitation.
- *Autologous blood injections:* In refractory cases, injections of 2 ml of autologous blood and 0.5 percent bupivicaine has been tried with good success in some centers.
- *Counterforce bracing (called the tennis elbow or forearm band):* These forces release the forces in the ECRB region.
- *Rehabilitative exercises:* These are wrist flexion, extension, forearm supination and pronation, wrist radial and ulnar deviations at three sets of ten repetitions everyday for 2–6 months is known to give good results.
- *Ultrasound-guided percutaneous needle therapy:* This consists of ultrasound-guided corticosteroid injection and needle debridement of the structures around lateral epicondyle.

Indications: In small tears, not responding to conservative therapy and if too small for surgery.

Advantages

- Minimally invasive procedure.
- Restoration of function is rapid.
- The option of surgery is still open.

In expert's hands, it has a success rate of 65 percent.

Quick facts

Significant relief of symptoms in tennis elbow:

• Changing tennis strokes	92 percent
• Stretching exercises	84 percent
• Use of splints	83 percent
• NSAIDs/steroid	85 percent
• Physiotherapy	50–75 percent
• Rest more than 1 month	72 percent

GOLFER'S ELBOW

(Syn: Epitrochleitis, Medial tennis elbow)

Did you know?

Golfer's elbow is also called Swimmer's elbow.

Definition

It is a tendinopathy of the insertion of the epitrochlear muscles [flexors of the fingers of the hand flexor carpi radialis (FCR) and pronators].

Epitrochleitis is very similar to lateral epicondylitis (tennis elbow) but occurs on the medial side of the elbow, where the pronator teres and the flexors of the wrist and fingers originate. Tensing of these muscles by resisted wrist and finger flexion in pronation will provoke the pain (Fig. 3.21).

Tenderness is often less well localized than in tennis elbow.

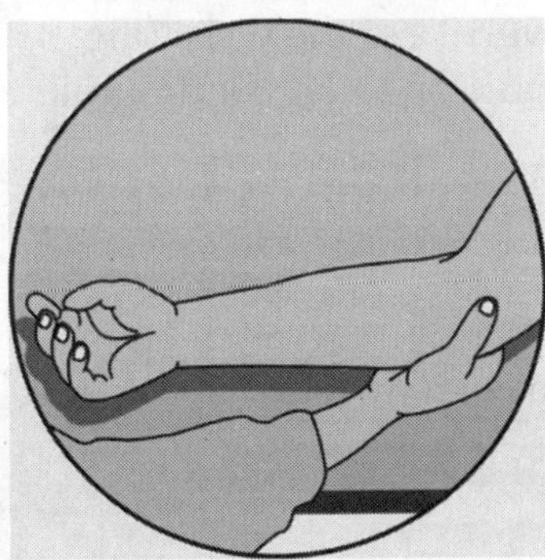

Fig. 3.21: Method of eliciting tenderness in Golfer's elbow

Do you know?

Tennis elbow is nine times more common than Golfer's elbow.

Treatment

It is the same as for tennis elbow, but the treatment is even less satisfactory.

Lesser-known but interesting elbow conditions

You know about tennis and Golfer's elbow, but do you know about:

Boxer's elbow: This is also called as hyperextension overload syndrome or olecranon impingement syndrome and is due to the repetitive valgus hyperextension by a boxer during jabbing.

Little leagues elbow: This is a medial epicondyle avulsion fracture. It is seen commonly in children and adolescents involved in throwing sports.

SPORTS INJURIES OF THE WRIST AND HAND

de QUERVAIN'S DISEASE

It is also called as stenosing tenosynovitis of the first dorsal compartment of the wrist involving the abductor pollicis longus and extensor pollicis brevis tendons.

Etiology

Exact cause is not known. de Quervain's disease is commonly seen in women between 30 and 50 years of age, and may be due to repeated overuse of the wrist (Fig. 3.22). Trigger finger is common in conditions like rheumatoid arthritis.

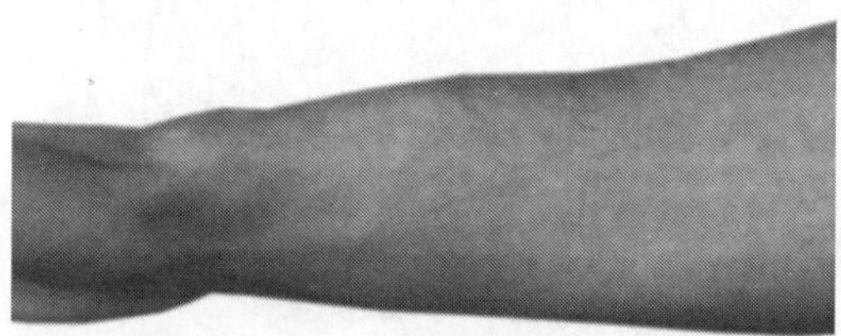

Fig. 3.22: Clinical photograph of de Quervain's disease

Clinical Features

Pain and limitation of the movements of the involved tendons are the presenting features. In this, the common sheath of abductor pollicis longus and extensor pollicis brevis tendons at the wrist are involved. Tenderness can be elicited by sudden ulnar deviation of the flexed hand [Finkelstein's test—with the thumb tucked inside the palm (Fig. 3.23)].

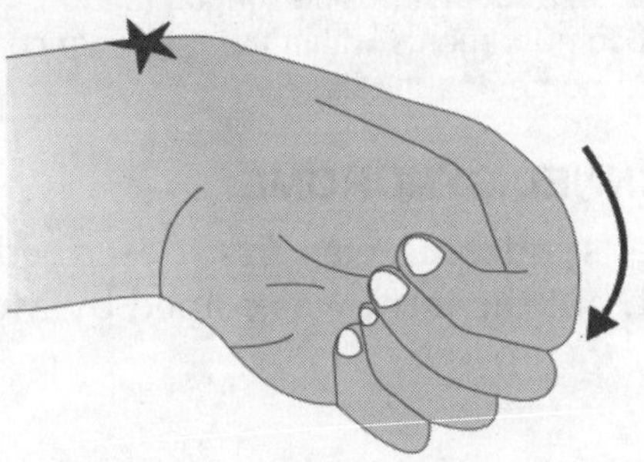

Fig. 3.23: Finkelstein's test

> **Pitfalls**
>
> **Do you know that Finkelstein's test is not pathognomonic of de Quervain's disease? It is also positive in:**
>
> - First carpomatacarpal arthritis.
> - Warrenberg's syndrome.
> - Arthritis of radiocarpal and intercarpal joints.
>
> **Interesting facts**
>
> Do you know about intersection syndrome? Well, it is tenosynovitis of the II dorsal compartment.

Treatment

Conservative Methods

This treatment consists of rest, NSAIDs, local infiltration of hydrocortisone, wrist immobilization, etc.

Surgery

Division of the appropriate retinaculum if the above measures fail.

> **Mystifying facts**
>
> **Do you know the reasons for failure of conservative treatment in de Quervain's disease?**
>
> - Anomalous tendons.
> - Multiple slips of abductor pollicis longus tendon.
> - Multiple subcompartments within the first wrist compartment. This is seen in 75 percent of the cases.

CARPAL TUNNEL SYNDROME

Carpal tunnel syndrome was first described by Sir James Paget in 1854, but the term was coined by Moerisch.

Anatomy

Bones bound the carpal tunnel on three sides and a ligament on one side (Fig. 3.24). The floor is an osseous arch formed by the carpal bones and the transverse carpal ligament forms the roof.

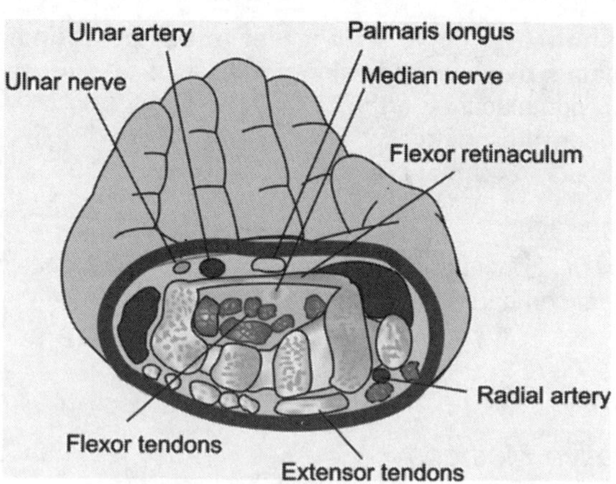

Fig. 3.24: Anatomy of the carpal tunnel

Contents

Tendons of flexor digitorum superficialis and pro-fundus in a common sheath, tendon of flexor pollicis longus in an independent sheath and the median nerve (Fig. 3.25).

Synovitis of the above tendons can generate pressure on the nerve.

Know that 9 tendons and 1 nerve pass through the carpal tunnel.

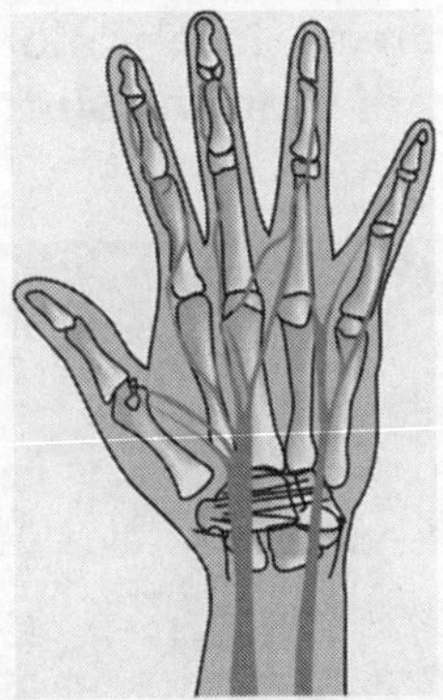

Fig. 3.25: Median nerve coursing through the carpal tunnel

Causes

General

Inflammatory—e.g. rheumatoid arthritis.

Endocrine—hypothyroidism, diabetes mellitus, menopause, pregnancy, etc. are some of the important endocrine causes.

Metabolic cause—gout.

Local

These cause crowding of the space. Malunited Colles' fracture, ganglion in the carpal region, osteoarthritis of the carpal bones, and wrist contusion, hematoma, etc. are some of the important local causes.

Remember

Mnemonic PRAGMATIC for causes of carpal tunnel syndrome [(*P*—Pregnancy, *R*—Rheumatoid arthritis, *A*—Arthritis degenerative, *G*—Growth hormone abnormalities (acromegaly), *M*—Metabolic (gout, diabetes myxoedema, etc.), *A—Alcoholism, T*—Tumors, *I*—Idiopathic, *C*—Connective tissue disorders (e.g. amyloidosis)].

Clinical Stages or Features (Figs 3.26A and B)

Stage I: In this stage, pain is usually the presenting complaint and the patient complains of characteristic discomfort in the hand, but there is no precise localization to the median nerve. There may be history of morning stiffness in the hand.

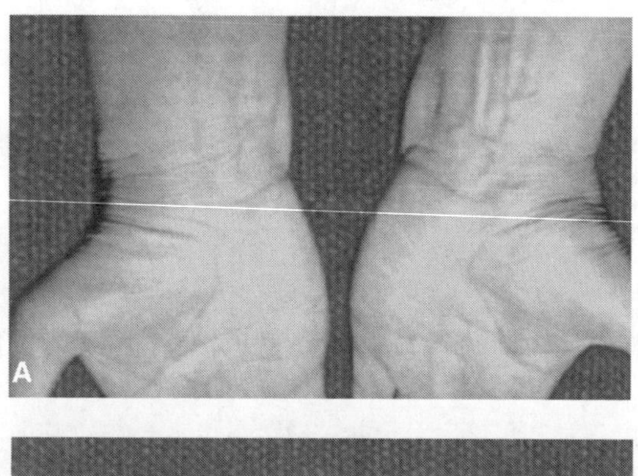

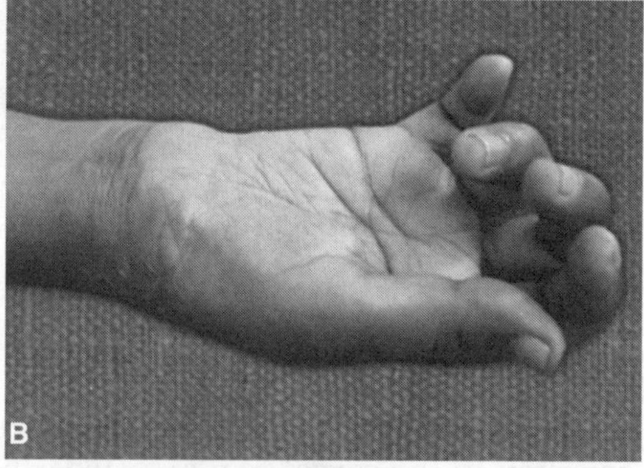

Figs 3.26A and B: (A) Clinical photograph of bilateral carpal tunnel syndrome, (B) Carpal tunnel (Clinical photo)

Stage II: In this stage, symptoms of tingling and numbness, pain, paresthesia, etc. are localized to areas supplied by the median nerve.

Stage III: Here, the patient complains of clumsiness in the hand and impairment of digital functions, etc.

Stage IV: In this stage, sensory loss in the median nerve distribution area can be elicited and there is obvious wasting of the thenar eminence.

Clinical Tests

These are provocative tests and act as important screening methods and as an adjunct to the electrophysiological testing.

Wrist flexion (Phalen's test): The patient is asked to actively place the wrist in complete but unforced flexion. If tingling and numbness are produced in the median nerve distribution of the hand within 60 seconds, the test is positive. It is the most sensitive provocative test (Fig. 3.27). It has a specificity of 80 percent.

Tourniquet test: A pneumatic blood pressure cuff is applied proximal to the elbow and inflated higher than the patient's systolic blood pressure. The test is positive if there is paresthesia or numbness in the region of median nerve distribution of the hand. It is less reliable and is specific in 65 percent of cases only.

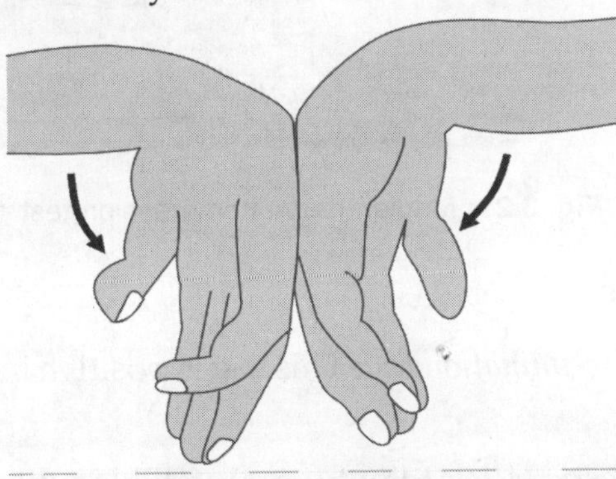

Fig. 3.27: Phalen's test

Median nerve percussion test: The examiner gently taps the median nerve at the wrist (Fig. 3.28). The test is positive if there is tingling sensation. Seen only in 45 percent of cases.

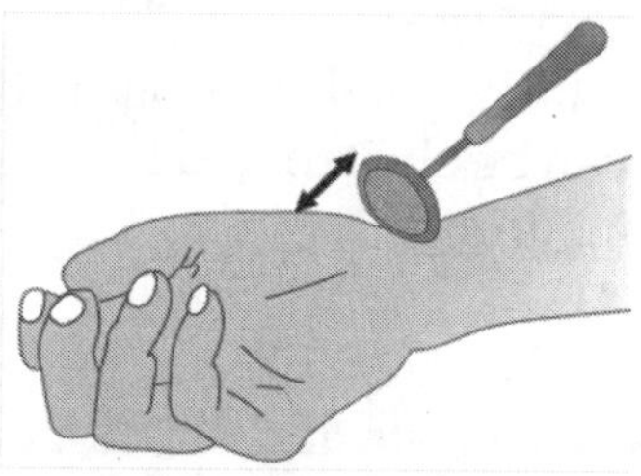

Fig. 3.28: Median nerve percussion test

Median nerve compression test: Direct pressure is exerted equally over both wrists by the examiner (Fig. 3.29). The first phase of the test is the time taken for symptoms to appear (15 sec to 2 min). The second phase is the time taken for the symptoms to disappear after release of pressure.

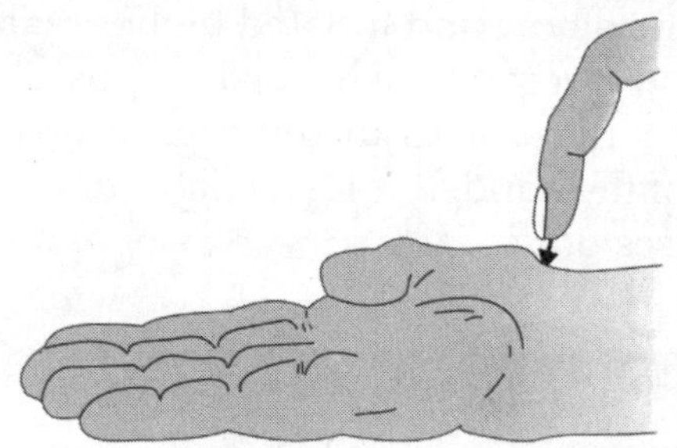

Fig. 3.29: Median nerve compression test

Other Tests

Two-point discrimination test: This test is positive in about one-third cases.

Electrodiagnostic tests are not very infallible with 10 percent individuals having normal values.

Treatment

Nonoperative methods: In the initial stages, non-steroidal anti-inflammatory drugs NSAIDs are given. If it is unsuccessful, steroids like prednisolone for 8 days starting with 40 mg for 2 days and tapering by 10 mg every 2 days are tried. Use of carpal tunnel splint is also advocated (Fig. 3.30).

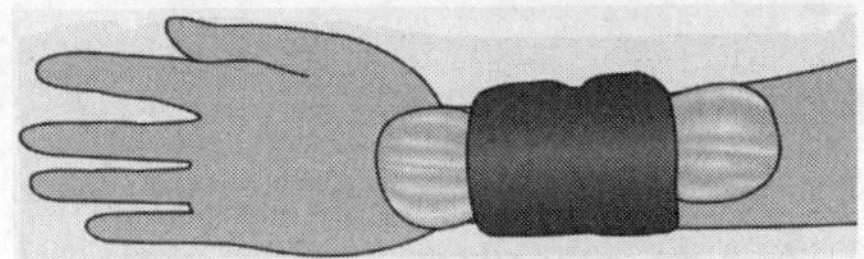

Fig. 3.30: Carpal tunnel splint

Injection treatment: This is indicated in patients with intermittent symptoms, duration of complaints less than one year and if there is no sensory deficits, no marked thenar wasting, etc.

In the injection therapy, a single infusion of cortisone with splinting for 3 weeks is tried.

Surgery: This consists of division of flexor retinaculum and transverse carpal ligament and is indicated in failed nonoperative treatment, thenaratrophy, sensory loss, etc. (Fig. 3.31).

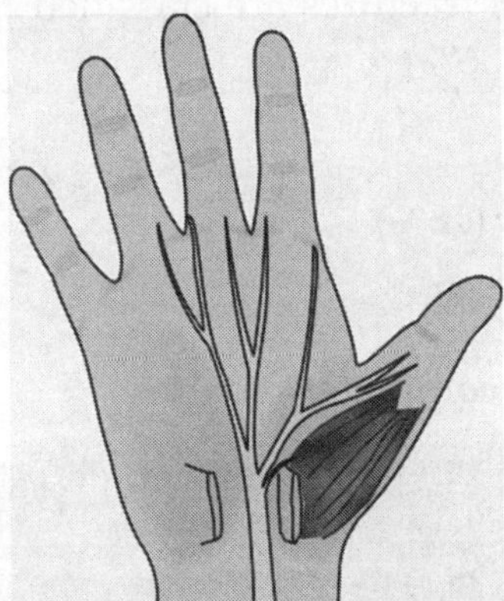

Fig. 3.31: Surgical division of the transverse carpal ligament

What is new in the treatment of carpal tunnel?

Chow's technique

This is an endoscopic release of the carpal ligament. It is a reliable alternative for the open procedure and has a success rate of 93.3 percent.

INJURIES TO THE PHALANX

DISTAL PHALANX FRACTURES

These fractures are usually caused by crushing injuries they are frequently comminuted.

Salient Features

- Very commonly injured.
- Soft tissue coverage is less.
- In nail bed injuries, hematoma can be seen through the nail bed.

Mechanism of Injury

It is mainly due to direct crush injuries. Indirect forces may result in avulsion injuries.

Classifications

Distal phalangeal fractures are classified into:

- Longitudinal (36%)
- Transverse
- Tuft (63%)
- Basal fractures (18%)
  - Dorsal
  - Volar
- Intra-articular complete fractures.

Do you know the difference between dorsal base and Mallet fracture?

- *Mallet fingers:* < 25 percent involvement of articular cartilage and hence stable.

- *Dorsal basal fractures:* > 25 percent involvement of articular cartilage and hence unstable.

Clinical Features

Pain, swelling, tenderness and deformity of the tip of the finger. Loss of function of the distal IP joints is seen.

Radiograph

Plain X-ray of the finger AP, lateral and oblique views help to make the diagnosis.

Treatment

Three modalities of treatment are described namely:

Conservative Method: This is reserved mainly for undisplaced, longitudinal and tuft fractures. The method employed is splinting for 3 to 4 weeks (Fig. 3.32).

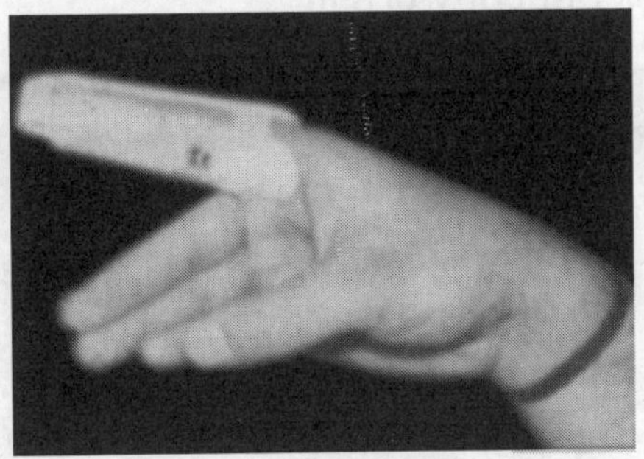

Fig. 3.32: Finger cot splint

Closed Reduction and Percutaneous Fixation:
This is reserved for:

- Transverse shaft fractures where external splinting fails to hold the fragments.
- Dorsal base fractures with > 25 percent involvement of articular surfaces. Here the K-wire pinning should be done across the DIP joint.

Open Reduction and Internal Fixation:
This is indicated in:

- Volar base fractures with disruption of the flexor digitorum profundus (FDP) insertion.
- Dorsal base fractures with 30 to 40 percent involvement of the articular surface.

MALLET FINGER (SYN: BASEBALL FINGER, DROP FINGER, CRICKET FINGER)

Mallet finger is a common injury usually due to forced flexion of the distal phalanx while the extensor tendons are actively trying to extend the finger (Fig. 3.33). The baseball catcher, football receiver and others are vulnerable to this injury. Depending upon whether the thin extensor tendon is torn in its substance or pulls off a small piece of bone at its insertion, two types are recognized:

- Mallet finger of tendon origin.
- Mallet finger of bony origin.

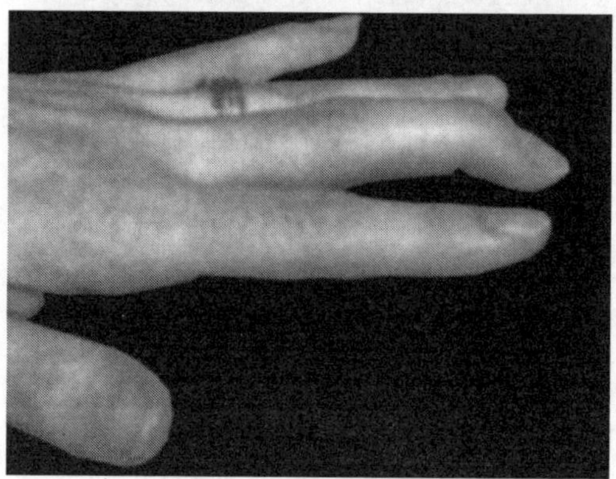

Fig. 3.33: Mallet finger (Clinical photo)

Tendon Origin

This is due to loss of extensor tendon continuity at the distal finger joint.

Mechanism of Injury

Here the end of the finger is forcibly flexed, when extensor tendon is taut, e.g. while tucking the bed, catching a ball, striking an object with extended finger, etc. (Figs 3.34A and B).

Clinical Features

Pain, swelling, tenderness, flexion deformity of the tip of the finger and inability of the patient to actively extend the finger at the distal PIP joint.

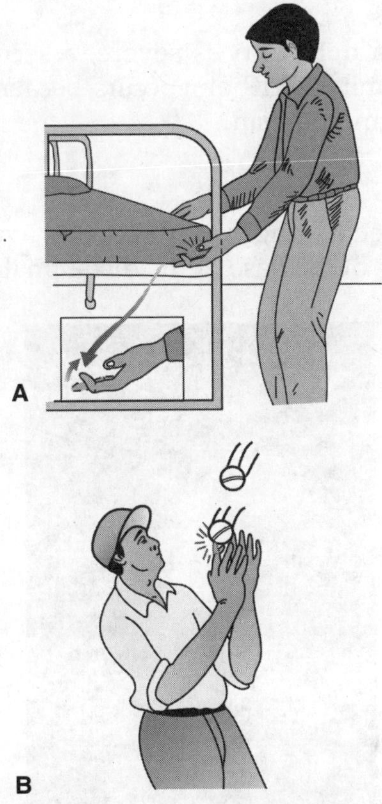

Figs 3.34A and B: Common mechanism of injury pertaining to mallet finger

Several Types

The following deformities could be seen based on the types of injuries.

- *Extensor tendon stretched* in this, degree of drop is less. There is loss of 5° to 20° of extension. There is weak active extension.
- *Extensor tendon ruptured* from its insertion into distal phalanx. There is 40° to 45° loss of extension. No active extension.
- *Avulsion fracture.* A small fragment of distal phalanx is avulsed with the extensor tendon. There is no active extension and it should be treated as tendon injuries rather than fractures.

If the flexion deformity is severe, a secondary hyper-extension deformity of PIP joint occurs, because of imbalance of the extensor mechanism.

Radiographs

X-ray of the affected finger may show an avulsion fracture of the dorsal lip of the base of the distal phalanx (Fig. 3.35).

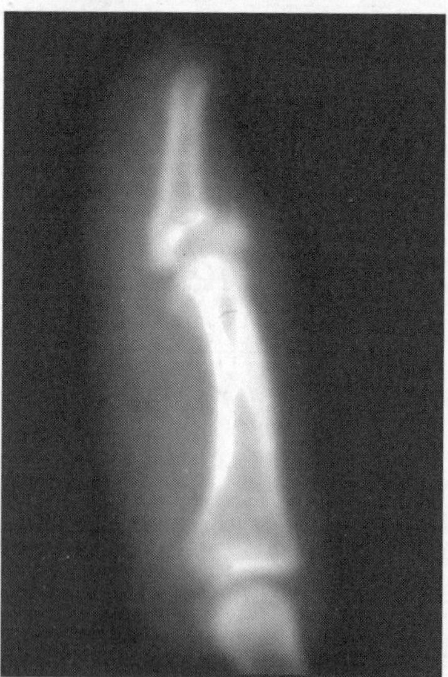

Fig. 3.35: Radiograph showing mallet fracture (Avulsion type)

Treatment

Nonoperative measures: This is reserved for pure dislocations, collateral ligament injuries and mallet finger. Various custom-made dorsal hyperextension splints (Mallet splints) are used for immobilizing the DIP joints.

Closed reduction and percutaneous fixation: This is reserved for mallet injuries in professionals like dentists, surgeons, sportspeople, etc. who cannot keep their fingers immobilized for long due to professional commitments.

Open reduction and internal fixation: This is indicated in the following situations:

- Avulsion of the profundus tendon and its reinsertion.
- Chronic subluxation of the DIP joint (> 3 weeks).
- Irreducible dislocations.

Mallet Finger of Bony Origin

This is less common. It is usually fixed with K-wire, if more than one-third of the dorsal articular surface is involved and if remainder of the distal phalanx is subluxated volar-wards.

Facts about Mallet Splints

In these cases, proximal interphalangeal joint of the finger is not immobilized but only the distal joint is immobilized by using:

a. Simple volar unpadded aluminum splint, which provides three-point pressure.
b. Dorsal padded aluminum splint.
c. A stack plastic mallet finger splint (Figs 3.36A and B).

Distal joint is put in slight hyperextension. The splint may cause pain and the amount of hyperextension should not cause blanching of the skin over DIP joint.

Splints are useful in cooperative patients, and in uncooperative patients. Smellie's cast is used. About 6 to 10 weeks of continuous immobilization is required. K-wire fixation is considered in patients like dentist or surgeon who wants to return to work quickly.

Lesser-Known but Important Thumb Injuries

- *Bowler's Thumb:* It is a traumatic neuropathy of the digital nerve of the thumb due to repeated friction from gripping a ball.
- *Gamekeeper's or Baseball Thumb:* This has been explained earlier.

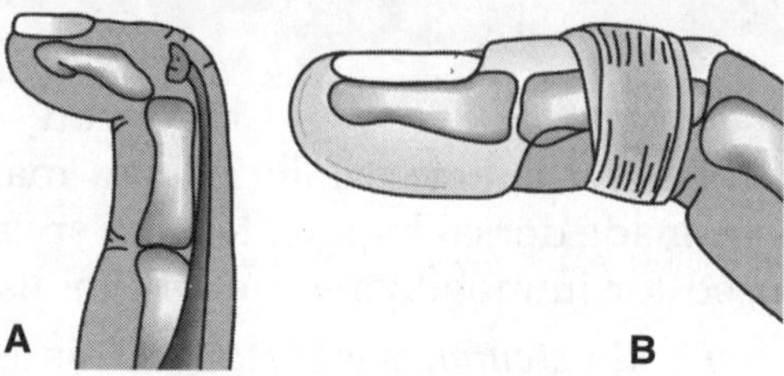

Figs 3.36A and B: (A) Mallet finger, and (B) Treatment by a dorsal splint

DISTAL INTERPHALANGEAL JOINT INJURIES

These injuries are usually due to ball catching sports.

Salient Features

- Pure dislocations without tendon ruptures are rare.
- Most of the times DIP joint dislocations are missed initially.
- Dislocation is mainly dorsal.
- Isolated injury to the collateral ligament and volar plate are rare.

Jersey finger: It is due to avulsion of flexor digitorum profundus from its insertion on distal phalanx. This is the opposite of 'mallet finger' and the patient is unable to flex the distal interphalangeal joint. It is seen in football and rugby players.

FRACTURES OF THE MIDDLE PHALANX

The three important injuries of special interest relating to the middle phalanx are:

- Isolated fracture of the volar base.
- Isolated fracture of the dorsal base.
- Pilon fractures. This consists of extensive metaphyseal comminution with involvement of the entire articular surfaces and bone loss.

All these injuries can pose problems in the management.

Clinical Features

Pain, swelling, tenderness, deformity of the finger and loss of finger functions are the usual complaints.

Radiographs

Plain X-ray of the finger AP, lateral and oblique views help to make the diagnosis.

Management

Volar Base Fractures

Nonoperative treatment: This consists of extension block splinting of the PIP joint and is indicated in volar base fractures with less than 40 percent involvement of the articular surface.

Closed reduction and internal fixation: This is indicated for both dorsal and volar base fractures of the middle phalanx with less than 40 percent articular surface involvement (Figs 3.37A and B).

Dynamic traction: This is a unique method of treatment and is indicated in volar base fractures of more than 40 percent and in the very difficult Pilon fractures.

Volar plate arthroplasty: This is indicated in chronic injuries and in volar base fractures greater than 40 percent.

Open reduction and internal fixations: This is indicated in single large fragment and in fixing bone graft to the metaphysis.

For dorsal base fractures, extension block pinning after closed reduction is the treatment of choice.

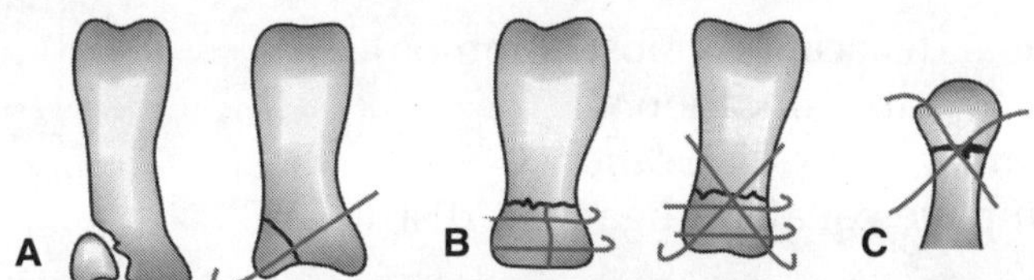

Figs 3.37A to C: Closed reduction and percutaneous fixation of various phalangeal fractures: (A) Unstable short oblique fractures, (B) Comminuted fracture, and (C) Condylar fracture

DISLOCATIONS OF THE IP JOINT

This could involve the proximal or distal interphalangeal joints.

Salient Features

- These are frequently missed.
- Common in ball catching sports.
- There is complete disruption of the collateral ligaments and the volar plate.
- About 50 percent cases occur in the middle finger followed by the ring finger.
- It is accompanied by gross swelling at the PIP joint.

Clinical Tests

Localized tenderness can be elicited by careful palpation of the PIP joint.

To test the integrity of the central slip: Instruct the patient to actively extend the PIP joint with the MP joint held in hyperextended position.

Tests to identify the development of Boutonnière deformity: Inability to passively flex the DIP joint while the PIP joint is held in extension heralds the onset of the Boutonnière deformity.

Stress tests: Lateral stress testing is performed with the fingers in complete extension and 30° of flexion. Greater than 20° of opening indicates complete tear of collateral ligaments.

Types

- Dorsal dislocation (most common).
- Pure volar dislocation.
- Rotatory volar dislocation.
- Complete collateral ligament disruption.

Clinical Features

Pain, swelling, tenderness and deformity. Loss of function of the distal IP joints is seen (Fig. 3.38).

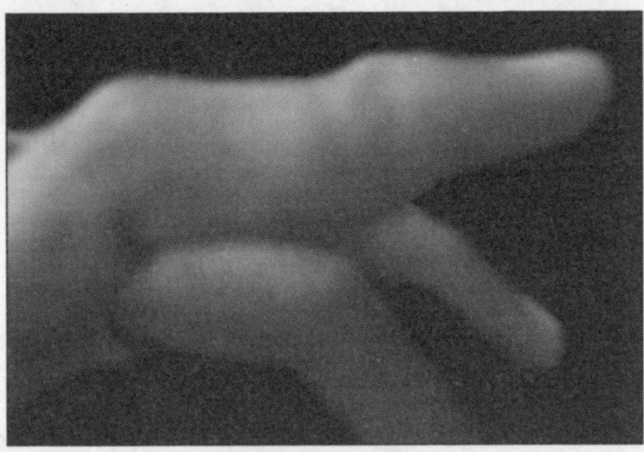

Fig. 3.38: Deformity as viewed from the sides (Clinical photo)

Radiographs

Plain X-ray of the finger AP, lateral and oblique views help to make the diagnosis.

Treatment

Nonoperative Management

This is indicated for closed injuries and for reducible injuries. After reduction:

- Buddy taping with immediate AROM for rotatory volar dislocation (Fig. 3.39).
- For collateral ligament injuries buddy taping with immediate AROM.
- For central slip disruption and volar dislocation, 4 to 6 weeks of PIP extension, splinting followed by a 2-week daytime dynamic splinting and a static night splinting. Throughout the period of splintage, DIP joint should be actively exercised (Fig. 3.40).
- Extension blocks splinting for 3 to 4 weeks for hyperextension injuries (dorsal dislocation).

Operative Management

Open reduction is indicated for open injuries, irreducible dislocations and injury to the collateral ligament of the index finger.

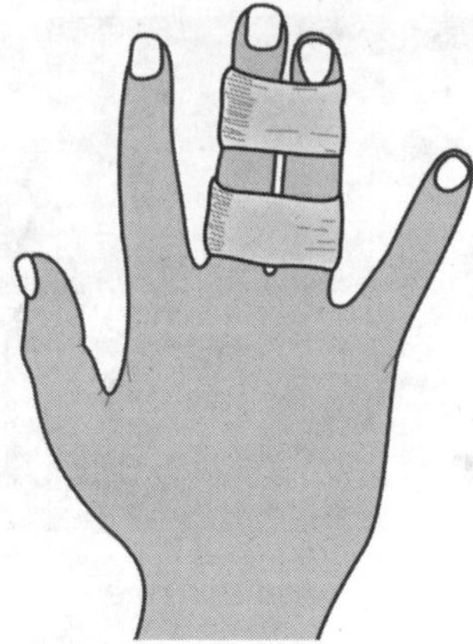

Fig. 3.39: Buddy taping

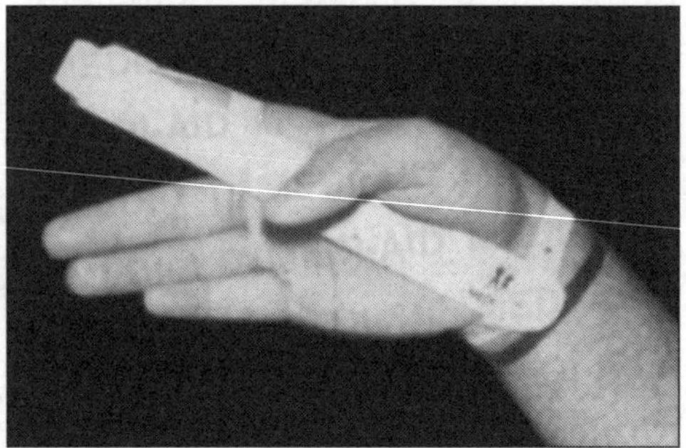

Fig. 3.40: Finger extension splint

PROXIMAL PHALANX FRACTURES

These are due to direct blow on the dorsum of fingers.

Salient Features

- Due to the deforming forces of the intrinsic muscles, transverse and short oblique fractures of the proximal phalanx angulate dorsally.
- The spiral and long oblique fractures shorten and rotate rather than angulate.
- Due to the action of FDS, fractures of the middle phalanx tend to angulate in either direction.

Classifications

- Head fractures—mainly intra-articular.
- Neck and shaft fractures—Extra-articular.
- Base—both extra-articular and intra-articular.

All these fractures could be:

- Minimally displaced but stable.
- Reducible but stable.
- Reducible but unstable.
- Irreducible.

Clinical Features

Pain, swelling, tenderness, deformity of the finger and loss of finger functions are the usual complaints.

Radiographs

Plain X-ray of the finger AP, lateral and oblique views helps to make the diagnosis (Fig. 3.41).

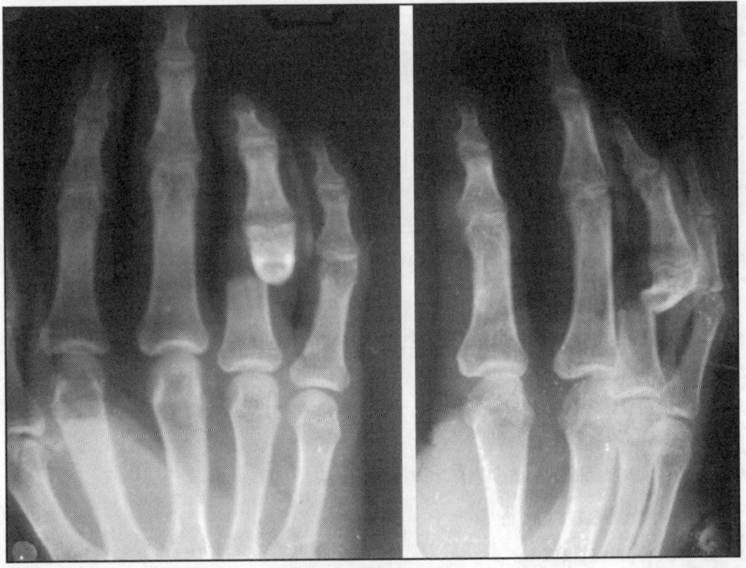

Fig. 3.41: Radiograph showing proximal phalanx fracture (Transverse)

Treatment Methods

Nonoperative Treatment

This is indicated for undisplaced and for reducible but stable extra-articular fractures. The methods employed are Buddy taping (Fig. 3.42) for undisplaced fractures and Burkhalter splint for the rest.

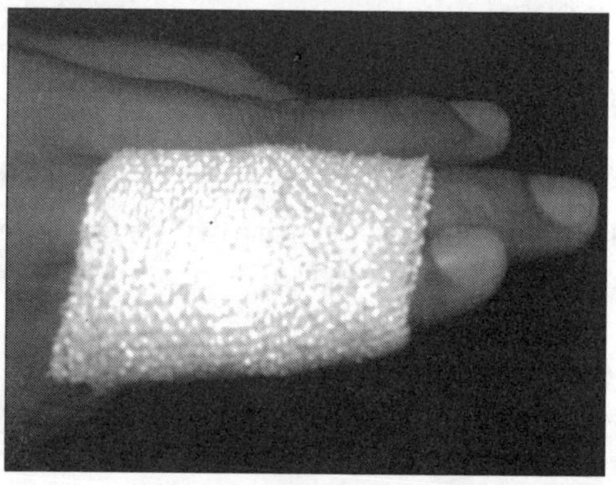

Fig. 3.42: Buddy taping

Closed Reduction and Percutaneous Fixation

This is reserved for transverse shaft fractures where external splinting fails to hold the fragments (Figs 3.43A and B).

Closed Reduction and Internal Fixation (IF)

This is indicated in the following situations:
- Oblique neck fracture.
- Reducible and stable intra-articular fracture of the middle phalanx.
- Reducible and unstable extra-articular fractures.

Open Reduction and Internal Fixation

This is indicated in:
- Open fractures
- Multiple fractures

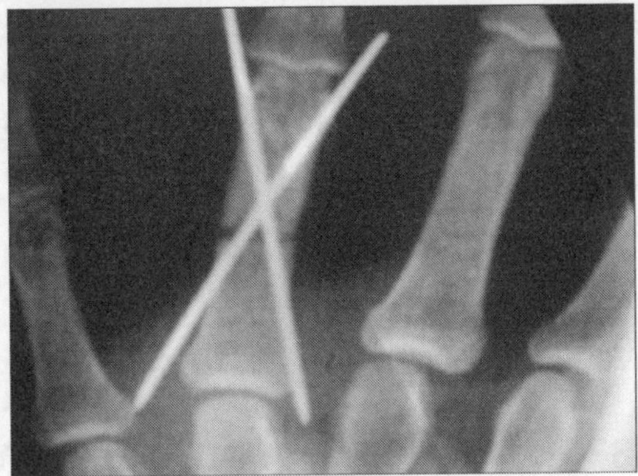

Fig. 3.43A: Radiograph showing proximal phalanx fracture fixed with criss cross K-wires

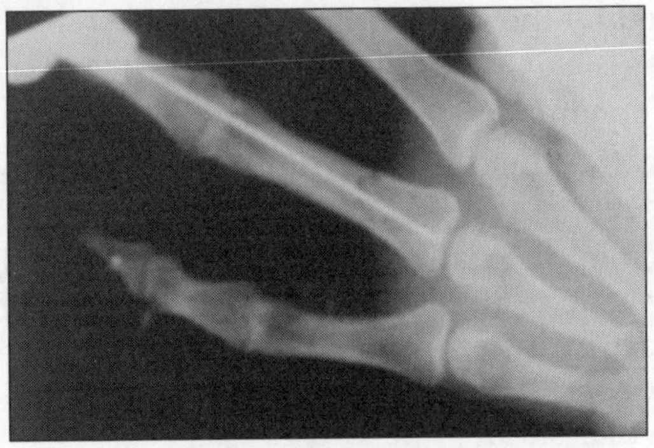

Fig. 3.43B: Radiograph showing K-wire fixation

- Soft tissue injury
- Intra-articular proximal phalanx fractures.

The options for internal fixation after open reduction are:

- Intraosseous wiring
- Composite wiring
- Screws only
- Plate and screw fixation.

The choice of the fixation depends on the experience and familiarity of the technique by the operating surgeon.

Complications of Phalangeal Fractures

Phalangeal fractures are very notorious to develop complications as the PIP joint is very less tolerant joint of the hand:

- Malunion
- Nonunion
- Stiffness
- Extension lags.

METACARPOPHALANGEAL JOINT DISLOCATIONS

Salient Features

- Dorsal dislocations are more common than volar.
- Small finger collateral ligament injuries are more common followed by the index finger.
- Dorsal dislocations are present with hyperextension deformity and are easy to reduce.
- During the dislocations, the volar plate does not get disturbed.
- Irreducible dislocations are called complex dislocations and are due to the volar plate entrapment. This is more common in index finger. Pathognomonic sign is the presence of sesamoid bones within the joint and puckering of the volar skin.
- Volar dislocations are very unstable but fortunately rare.

Clinical Features

Pain, swelling, tenderness over the MCP joint and loss of the affected finger and hand functions are the usual complaints.

Radiographs

Plain X-ray of the hand AP, lateral and oblique views help to make the diagnosis (Fig. 3.44).

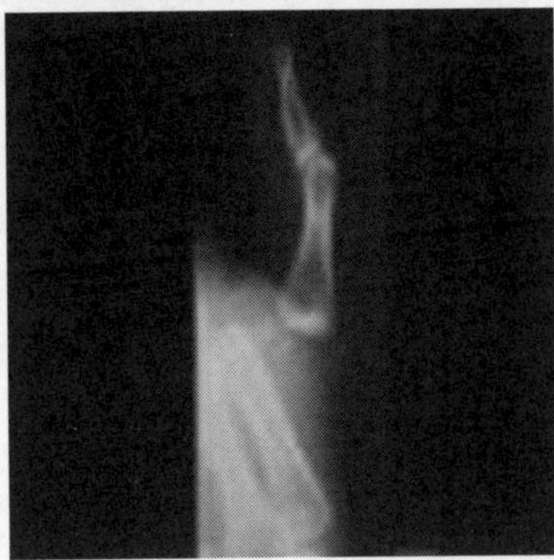

Fig. 3.44: Radiograph showing dislocation of 1st MCP joint

Treatment

Nonoperative Treatment

This is indicated in simple dorsal dislocations and collateral ligament ruptures. Reduction methods include:

- Flex the wrist to relax the flexor tendons.
- Apply firm but not excessive longitudinal tractions along the finger.
- Now gently flex the joint to achieve reduction.

The fingers are immobilized in Jones position as the digits are buddy taped.

Operative Treatment

This is indicated in complex dorsal dislocations, volar dislocation and radial collateral ligament injury of the index finger. The procedure consists of open reduction followed by repair or reconstruction of the collateral ligaments.

KAPLAN'S LESION

This is a complex irreducible dorsal metacarpophalangeal (MP) dislocation of fingers. Kaplan described buttonholing of the metacarpal head into the palm. Here there is an interposition of volar plate between the base of the proximal phalanx and the head of the metacarpal (Fig. 3.45).

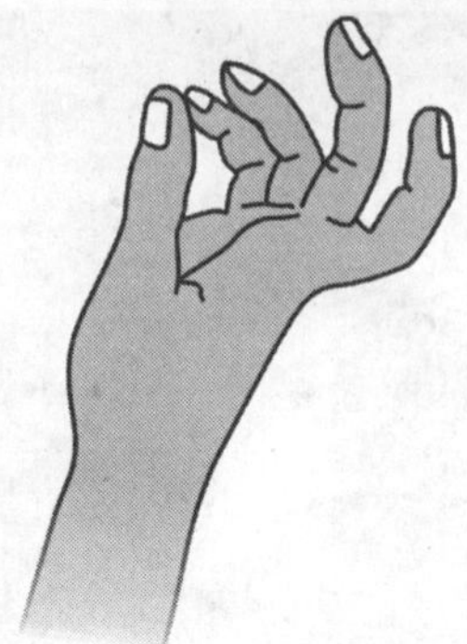

Fig. 3.45: Dislocation of II MP joint (Kaplan's lesion)

Incidence: This is commonly seen in the index finger next is thumb, little finger. It is rarely seen in long and ring fingers. Two types of dorsal dislocation occur in MP joints:

Simple: This can be reduced by closed methods.

Complex: This is irreducible and usually requires open reduction.

Both results from hyperextension injuries and in both the volar plate are torn at its proximal insertion into the metacarpal neck.

Clinical Features

Pain, swelling, hyperextension deformity at the MCP joint, tenderness over the dorsum of the hand and loss of the hand functions are the usual complaints (Figs 3.46A and B).

Radiographs

Plain X-ray of the hand AP, lateral and oblique views helps to make the diagnosis (Fig. 3.46C).

Diagnostic Clues

There are three clinical and radiographic clues to diagnosis:

- The metacarpophalangeal joint is only slightly hyper-extended, and the interphalangeal joint is flexed. In the

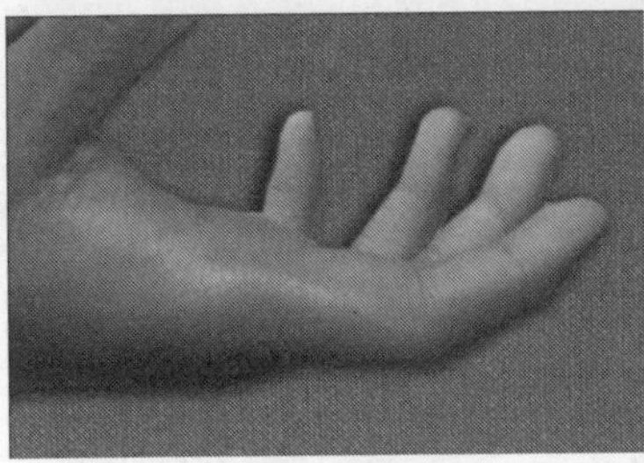

Fig. 3.46A: Kaplan's lesion (Clinical photo)

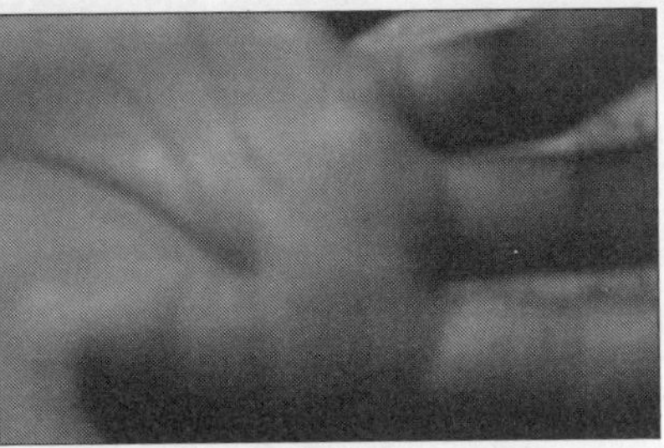

Fig. 3.46B: Volar view showing the puckered skin (Clinical photo)

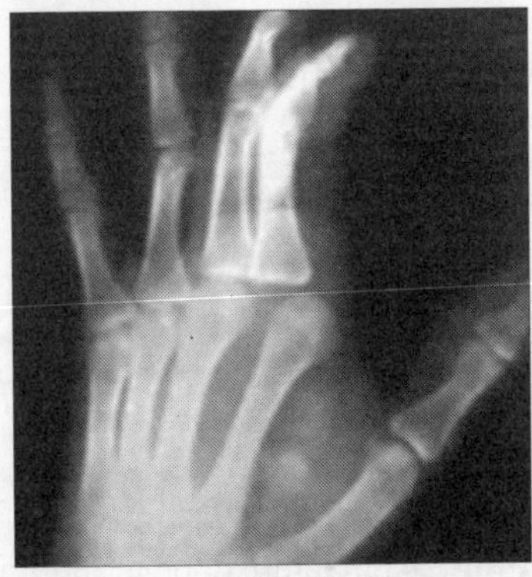

Fig. 3.46C: Radiograph of Kaplan's lesion

radiographs, proximal phalanx and metacarpals are nearly parallel.
- A constant finding is puckering of the volar skin, which is more readily seen in thumb than index finger.
- Pathognomonic radiographic sign is the presence of a sesamoid bone within a widened joint space. This is normally present with volar plate.

Treatment

A single attempt at closed reduction is made; and if this fails, surgical reduction either by the volar (Kaplan's operation) approach or by the dorsal approach is done.

Note: The single most important element preventing reduction in a complex metacarpophalangeal dislocation is interposition of volar plate within the joint.

DISLOCATION OF THE THUMB METACARPOPHALANGEAL JOINT (GAMEKEEPER'S THUMB, SKIER'S THUMB)

Injury to the ulnar collateral ligament of the first metacarpophalangeal (MP) joint is very common but a complete dislocation is rare. It heals with some residual instability (Fig. 3.47).

Diagnosis is made by direct palpation and stress tests. Treatment is by operative or nonoperative methods.

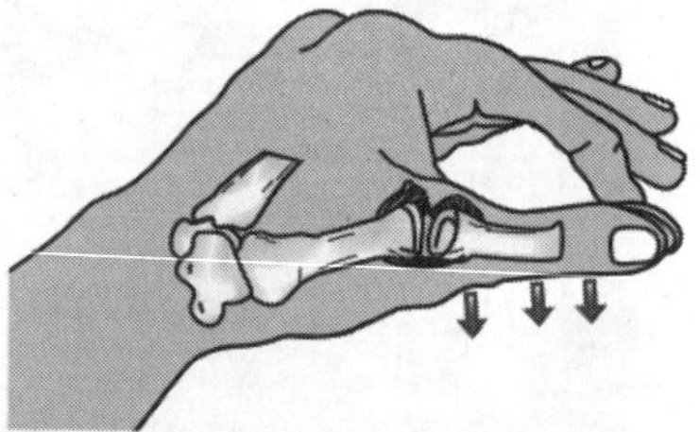

Fig. 3.47: Gamekeeper's thumb

INJURIES TO METACARPAL BONES

Metacarpal shaft fracture the common causes for these injuries are direct hit on the dorsum of the hand as in assault, boxing, fall, road traffic accident (RTA), etc. These fractures should be accurately reduced with no rotational malalignment and immobilized with either plaster (common) or percutaneous or open K-wire fixation (less common).

METACARPAL FRACTURE OF FINGERS

Salient Features

- The normal neck shaft angle in the metacarpal is 15°.
- A typical apex dorsal angulation is seen in transverse metacarpal neck and shaft fractures.

- This angulation is compensated clinically by a hyper-extension deformity.
- Spiral and oblique fractures tend to shorten and rotate than angulate.
- Rotational malalignment is not acceptable more than 10º.
- Due to the overlapping bone shadows, special X-ray views, as the Brewerton view is required. (Reverse oblique views and the Skyline views are other special views.)
- Metacarpals are responsible for the formation of the following three arches of the hand:
  - Transverse arch at the carpometacarpal joints.
  - Transverse arch at the MP joints.
  - A longitudinal broad convex dorsal arch.

These arches are maintained by:

- The interosseous ligaments at the bases.
- Deep transverse intermetacarpal ligaments distally:
  - Volar aspect of the neck of the metacarpal is the weakest point.
  - Intrinsic muscles are the primary deforming forces, which can be neutralized by MP joint flexion.
  - Reduction can be achieved by longitudinal traction and by flexion of the PIP joint.

Clinical Features

Pain, swelling, tenderness over the dorsum of the hand and loss of the hand functions are the usual complaints (Figs 3.48).

Radiographs

Plain X-ray of the hand AP, lateral and oblique views helps to make the diagnosis (Figs 3.49A and B).

Treatment Methods

Nonoperative treatment: This is indicated in the following situations:

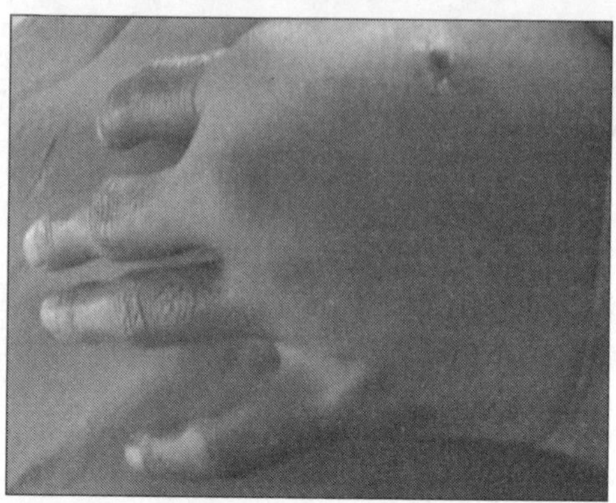

Fig. 3.48: Deformity and pin point compound (Clinical photo)

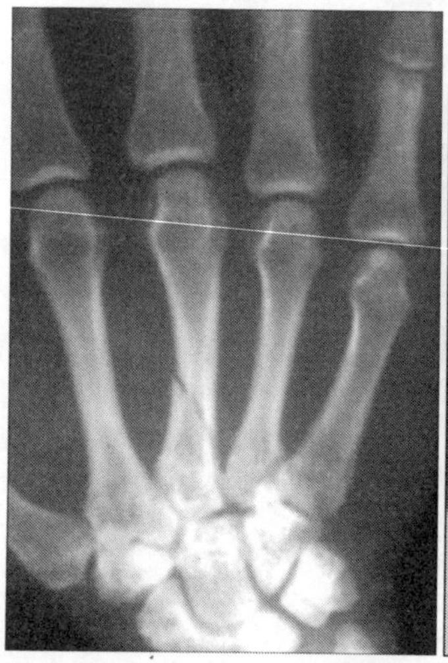

Fig. 3.49A: Radiograph showing oblique metacarpal fracture

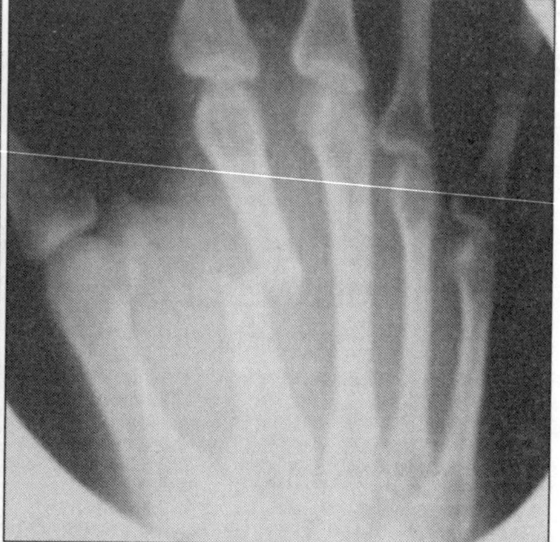

Fig. 3.49B: Radiograph showing transverse midshaft fracture

- Undisplaced fractures.
- Stable fractures (These have < 50 percent displacement, < 40° angulation and fracture obliquity of < 60°).

Methods: The hand can be immobilized by:

- Burk halter splint: This is ideal and is known to give good splints.

- Compression glove for 2 weeks.
- Hand-based cast is also effective and permits the patient to return to the work early.

Closed Reduction and Internal Fixation

This is indicated for fractures that are unstable after reduction and for base fractures. This is mainly used for extra-articular fractures but can also be used for intra-articular fractures that are stable with K-wire fixation alone after reduction.

Open Reduction and Internal Fixation

This is indicated in the following:

- Multiple fractures
- Open fractures
- Irreducible fractures
- Displaced intra-articular fractures.

The choice of the method of internal fixation devices could be:

- Intramedullary fixation through a Steinmann's pin, multiple prebent K-wires, etc.
- Screws only
- Plate and screws
- Intraosseous wiring
- Composite wiring.

The choice of fixation should be the one with which the surgeon is most familiar with (Figs 3.50A to C).

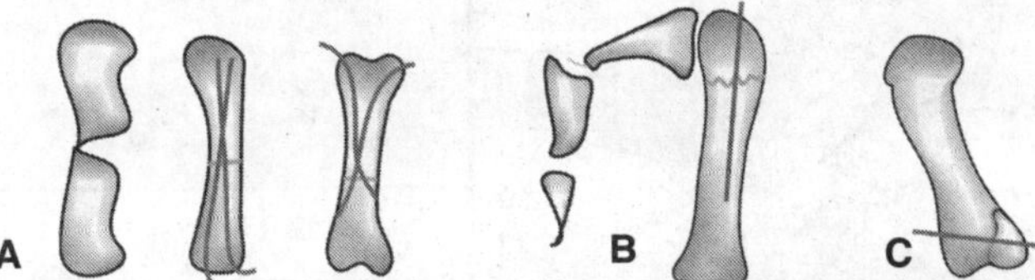

Figs 3.50A to C: Metacarpal fractures treated by closed reduction and percutaneous pinning: (A) Unstable fracture fixed with criss-cross K-wires, (B) Neck fracture fixed by intramedullary fixation, (C) Bennett's fracture fixed with K-wire

External Fixations

This is reserved for comminuted intra-articular fractures of the base of the fifth metacarpal bone where internal fixation is not suitable.

Complications

- Nonunion
- Avascular necrosis in periarticular fractures.
- Angular malunion
- Rotational malunion
- Intra-articular malunion
- Stiffness of the fingers.

METACARPAL FRACTURE OF THE LITTLE FINGER (BOXER'S FRACTURE)

When a boxer punches the jaw of his opponent with his fist and wins the bout, his ecstasy may be shortlived when he finds his little finger is broken, what he has actually broken is the neck of the fifth metacarpal bone and this is due to a direct impact on the dorsum of the hand (Fig. 3.51A).

Mechanism of Injury

This injury is also seen in assaults, RTAs, fall, etc.

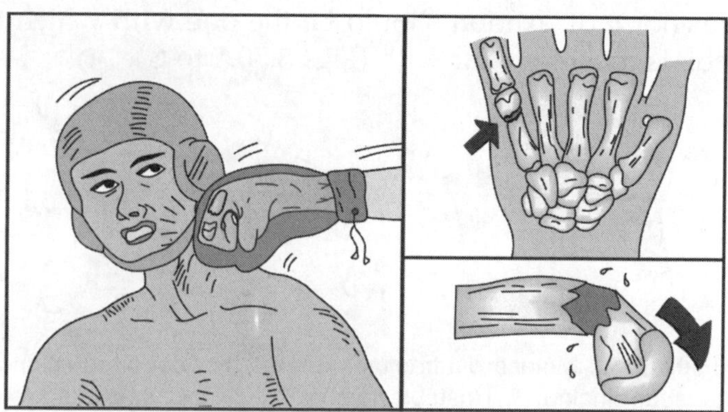

Fig. 3.51A: Mechanism of injury in boxer's fracture

Clinical Features

Patient may present with pain, swelling, tenderness over the dorsum of the ulnar border of the hand.

Radiographs

Plain X-ray of the hand AP, lateral and oblique views helps to make the diagnosis (Fig. 3.51B).

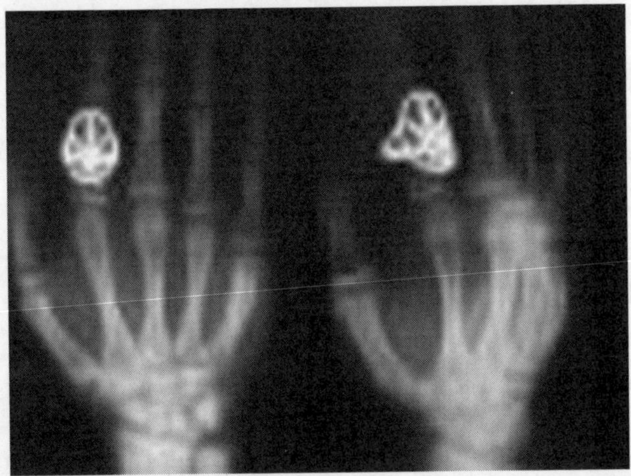

Fig. 3.51B: Radiograph showing boxer fracture

Treatment

These fractures need to be accurately reduced with no rotational malalignment. Closed reduction and fixation with either plaster cast or percutaneous K-wire fixation can do this.

METACARPAL HEAD FRACTURES

These are also known as *'fight bite'* fractures as they occur when the patient strikes an opponent's teeth in a fist fight. The clinical presentation and the investigations are the same as for metacarpal neck fractures. They are frequently intra-articular and need open reduction and internal fixation with K-wire.

METACARPAL FRACTURE OF THE THUMB

Salient Features

- Most of the thumb metacarpal fractures are intra-articular at the carpometacarpal joint.
- The volar beak of basal fracture is not palpable.
- Special X-ray views consisting of true AP and lateral views are required.
- Basal fractures of the thumb are divided into:
  –Extra-articular fractures: Transverse/oblique.
  –Partial articular fracture (Bennett's).
  –Total articular fracture (Rolando).

INJURIES OF THE CARPOMETACARPAL JOINTS OF THE THUMB

Introduction

Carpometacarpal joints act as a link between the wrist and hand. The joints of the index and middle fingers are stable while that of the thumb and the little fingers are more mobile. Thumb carpometacarpal dislocations are more common and are dealt here. The two important dislocations are Bennett's fracture dislocation and Rolando fracture dislocation.

BENNETT'S FRACTURE

Bennett's fracture is a fracture dislocation of the palmar base of the first metacarpal bone of the thumb with either subluxation or dislocation of the first carpometacarpal joint.

Edward Bennett described it in 1882. It is an intra-articular fracture.

Mechanism of Injury

The common mechanism of injury is an axial blow directed against the partially flexed metacarpal, in most cases during "fist fights".

Characteristics of this Fracture

- Fracture line separates major part of the metacarpal from a small volar lip fragment producing disruption of the carpometacarpal joint.
- It is an avulsion rather than a pure dislocation. It occurs because of strong anterior oblique ligament.
- Size of the volar lip fragment and amount of shaft displacement vary.

Displacing muscle Forces in the Bennett's Fracture

- At the distal fragment, it is the adductor pollicis muscle.
- At the proximal fragment, it is the abductor pollicis longus muscle.

Base of the thumb metacarpal is pulled dorsally and medially by the abductor pollicis longus (Fig. 3.52), while the distal attachment of adductor further levers the base into abduction.

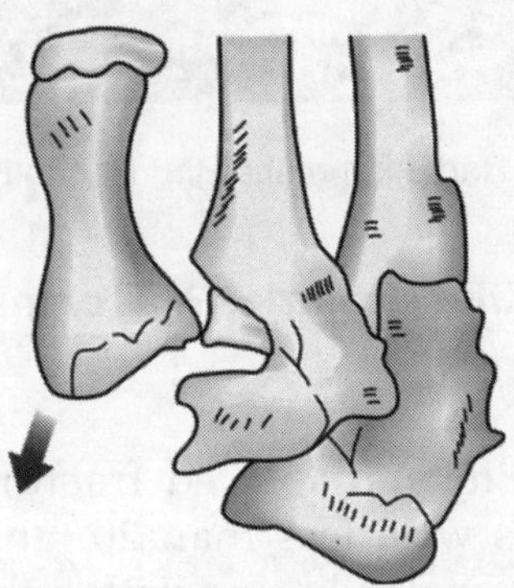

Fig. 3.52: Bennett's fracture. Thick arrow indicates the line of pull of abductor policis longus

How do they present? Clinical Features

The patient complains of

- Pain,
- Swelling and
- Tenderness over the base of the thumb.
- Movements of the thumb are severely restricted.

Radiograph

Plain X-rays of the hand help to make the diagnosis of the fracture accurately (Fig. 3.53).

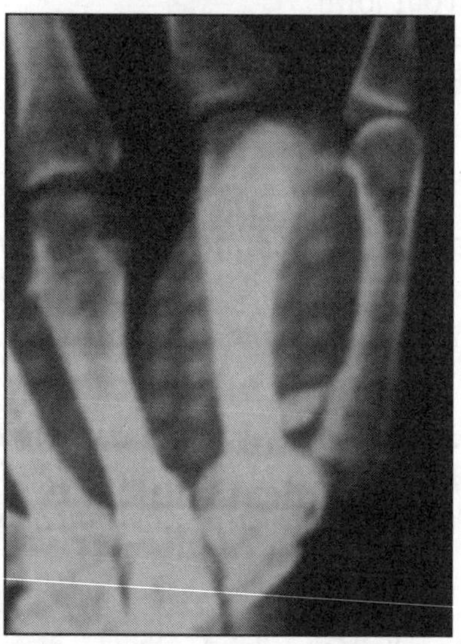

Fig. 3.53: Radiograph showing Bennett's fracture

How to manage these injuries? Treatment

Nonoperative Methods

This is indicated in undisplaced fractures and in extra-articular fractures with less than 20° angulation. Closed reduction and external splinting with a thumb spica is the treatment method of choice.

Surgery

Percutaneous fixation Methods: A single attempt at closed reduction is tried first and a percutaneous fixation with K-wire is usually performed.

Open reduction: If it fails, ORIF with K-wire or a small screw is carried out.

ROLANDO FRACTURE

Introduction

Rolando fractures are comminuted intra-articular fractures of the base of the thumb. Presentation and management are similar to Bennett's fracture.

How does it present? Clinical Features

- Pain,
- Swelling,
- Tenderness over the dorsum of the thumb and
- Loss of the thumb functions are the usual complaints.

Radiograph

Plain X-ray of the thumb AP, lateral and oblique views helps to make the diagnosis.

How to manage this fracture? Treatment Methods

Nonoperative Methods

This is indicated in undisplaced fractures and in extra-articular fractures with less than 20° angulation. Closed reduction and external splinting with a thumb spica is the treatment method of choice.

Closed Reduction and Internal Fixation

This is indicated in:

- Bennett's fracture.
- Rolando fracture.
- Oblique extra-articular fracture.

Open Reduction and Internal Fixation

This is indicated in uncomminuted Rolando fracture and irreducible Bennett's fracture.

External Fixations

This is indicated in highly comminuted Rolando fracture where internal fixation is contraindicated.

Index

Clinical Notes

Clinical Notes

Clinical Notes

Clinical Notes

Clinical Notes

Clinical Notes